The Menopause Maze

of related interest

Eat to Get Younger
Tackling Inflammation and Other Ageing
Processes for a Longer, Healthier Life
Lorraine Nicolle and Christine Bailey
ISBN 978 1 84819 179 2
eISBN 978 0 85701 125 1

Sleep Better with Natural Therapies
A Comprehensive Guide to Overcoming Insomnia,
Moving Sleep Cycles and Preventing Jet Lag
Peter Smith
ISBN 978 1 84819 182 2
eISBN 978 0 85701 140 4

Vital Face
Facial Exercises and Massage for Health and Beauty
Leena Kiviluoma
ISBN 978 1 84819 166 2
eISBN 978 0 85701 130 5

Make Yourself Better
A Practical Guide to Restoring Your Body's
Wellbeing through Ancient Medicine
Philip Weeks
ISBN 978 1 84819 012 2
eISBN 978 0 85701 077 3

Recovery and Renewal
Your Essential Guide to Overcoming Dependency
and Withdrawal from Sleeping Pills, Other
'Benzo' Tranquillisers and Antidepressants
Revised Edition
Baylissa Frederick
ISBN 978 1 84905 534 5
eISBN 978 0 85700 964 7

THE MENPAUSE MAZE

THE COMPLETE GUIDE TO CONVENTIONAL, COMPLEMENTARY AND SELF-HELP OPTIONS

DR MEGAN A. ARROLL AND LIZ EFIONG

FOREWORD BY DR JOHN MORAN

SINGING
DRAGON
LONDON AND PHILADELPHIA

First published in 2016
by Singing Dragon
an imprint of Jessica Kingsley Publishers
73 Collier Street
London N1 9BE, UK
and
400 Market Street, Suite 400
Philadelphia, PA 19106, USA

www.singingdragon.com

Library of Congress Cataloging in Publication Data
Names: Arroll, Megan A., author. | Efiong, Liz, author.
Title: The menopause maze : the complete guide
to conventional, complementary
    and self-help options / Megan A. Arroll, Liz Efiong.
Description: London ; Philadelphia : Singing Dragon, 2016. | Includes
    bibliographical references and index.
Identifiers: LCCN 2015045670 | ISBN 9781848192744 (alk. paper)
Subjects: LCSH: Menopause--Treatment--Popular
works. | Menopause--Alternative
    treatment--Popular works. | Menopause--Nutritional aspects--Popular works.
    | Menopause--Diet therapy--Popular works. | Self-care, Health
Classification: LCC RG186 .A77 2016 | DDC 618.1/75--dc23
LC record available at http://lccn.loc.gov/2015045670

British Library Cataloguing in Publication Data
A CIP catalogue record for this book is available from the British Library

ISBN 978 1 84819 274 4
eISBN 978 0 85701 221 0

Printed and bound in the United States

CONTENTS

Acknowledgements 6

Foreword 7

Disclaimer 9

Preface 10

Chapter 1   Overview and the Experience of the Menopause . 13

Chapter 2   Basic Principles for Hormonal Health 48

Chapter 3   Nutrition and Dietary Supplements for the
            Menopause 69

Chapter 4   Psychological and Behavioural Interventions 90

Chapter 5   Complementary and Alternative Medicine
            (CAM) Therapies 108

Chapter 6   Self-help 126

Chapter 7   Bioidentical and Non-Bioidentical Hormone
            Therapy: History and Controversies 146

Chapter 8   What Type of HRT is Right for Me? 176

Chapter 9   Medical Management 196

Chapter 10 Pulling it All Together 221

Useful Addresses/Websites 228

Endnotes 230

Index 251

ACKNOWLEDGEMENTS

Megan and I both realised there was a need for a 'Complete Guide' on the menopause at the end of 2013. Although I had read, researched and written extensively on the subject of hormones and health, when it came to my own personal experience of the menopause, I found I still lacked quality, evidence-based information to enable me to make informed decisions. There didn't seem to be a single text that covered conventional, complementary and self-help options in one book. I knew Megan also had a keen interest in women's health and so the idea of *The Menopause Maze* was born.

We are especially grateful to Dr John Moran, for reviewing the book, for his helpful comments and writing the foreword, not to mention answering my endless emails. Our thanks also to Professor Marc L'Hermite, for so generously replying to emails and reviewing the book. To our other reviewers Niki and Fiona, and to Kathy Whyte, friend and Artiste Extraordinaire, for her help with Figure 1. Last, but by no means least, our thanks go to Jane Evans, Kerrie Morton, and the team at Jessica Kingsley Publishers for sharing our vision and making it a reality.

FOREWORD

Megan A. Arroll and Liz Efiong have written a very comprehensive guide to the menopause. The information given should make it easier and less confusing to make an informed decision on what action to take.

The menopause is a time of change both mentally and physically, as well as spiritually. It is a time of life when a woman needs to stand back, take a deep breath and realise that she has at least another 30 years of good living to do and needs to move forward in a positive way. Quality of life is one of the most important aspects to consider.

The choices of what to do are many. In this very relevant book on the menopause, the authors review the many different and complex choices that women have to make. What I like about the book is the detail on the risks and benefits of hormone replacement therapy (HRT) and bioidentical hormone replacement therapy (BHRT), and all the scientific references that will allow a woman to make an informed choice. For women who need a summary of and take home messages on breast cancer risk and the benefits for the cardiovascular, skin, hair, bladder and vaginal health, the book gives easily accessible evidence-based guidance.

It is timely that NICE guidelines on the menopause and the treatment options have recently been published, and

GPs and doctors will have more information on how to help women at this time of life.

The authors have written a good guide to options other than conventional HRT. It is important to understand the differences between HRT and BHRT and consider what treatment the individual woman prefers for herself. As well as treating the symptoms of the menopause, the book explains how to reduce the risk of heart disease and osteoporosis, using nutrition as well as HRT.

Women need to remain active and well with a good quality of life during and after the menopause. The authors have written a detailed guide on how to do this.

Dr John Moran, Medical Director of Holistic Medical Clinic
and Specialist in Menopause and Nutritional Medicine

DISCLAIMER

Every effort has been made to ensure that the information contained in this book is correct, but it should not in any way be substituted for medical advice. Readers should always consult a qualified medical practitioner before adopting any complementary or alternative therapies. Neither the author nor the publisher takes responsibility for any consequences of any decision made as a result of the information contained in this book.

PREFACE

If you are reading this book, we would guess that you are either experiencing the menopause or wanting to prepare yourself for it. Around one third of a woman's life is lived after the menopause and after the menopause women become vulnerable to associated health conditions, such as heart disease, osteoporosis, and cognitive decline. In this book we cover preventative steps you can take to minimise your risks of these and other conditions.

Although the menopause is a natural milestone in women's lives and not a disease, it can have some unpleasant symptoms. The good news is that there are things you can do to improve your symptoms and your quality of life during and after the menopause. Fortunately, gone are the times when women had to suffer in silence through the menopause. Women today are much more informed than our mothers and grandmothers were and we have a wealth of information available to us – almost an information overload – but most of us lack the time to read it all. The internet is a wonderful resource but unfortunately it can be full of contradictory, and often incorrect, information.

There are many different options to help you deal with menopausal symptoms and we believe that every woman should be well-informed of the different options available in order to make a balanced choice. This is an ideal time of life to really assess your health so you can be in the best possible health in the future.

This book is timely as many of the major menopause societies around the world have updated their guidelines in the last few years, which we have included in the 'take home messages', which summarise the latest information and expert opinions throughout the book. 18th October 2015 was International Menopause Day. The International Menopause Society marked the day by publishing a report encouraging women to have a 'health audit' at menopause, and to make any necessary changes which will benefit their future wellbeing.

How to get the most out of this book

Chapter 1 gives you an overview of the physiology of menopause, including symptoms and impact on life, and risk factors for associated health issues, many of which are modifiable. Reducing risk factors is covered throughout the book.

Chapter 2 covers basic principles for health, including dietary and environmental factors, and the top ten health recommendations from the World Cancer Research Fund/ American Institute for Cancer Research.

Chapter 3 discusses diet, supplements and herbs that can be used to alleviate the symptoms of the menopause.

Chapter 4 covers the importance of reducing stress levels, and psychological therapies and stress reduction techniques that have been studied in relation to menopause, such as cognitive behavioural therapy (CBT) and mindfulness/ meditation.

Chapter 5 covers the research evidence on non-dietary complementary therapies such as yoga, acupuncture and reflexology and a guide to finding a reputable Complementary and Alternative Medicine (CAM) practitioner.

Chapter 6 covers self-help techniques, such as meditation/ stress management, exercise, and social support.

Chapter 7 covers what HRT is, how it works, the difference between bioidentical and non-bioidentical HRT, benefits and risks, and 'what the experts say'.

Chapter 8 should help you decide if HRT is right for you and, if so: what type, how to take it, and when to start/stop.

Chapter 9 covers non-hormonal medications that may be an option if HRT is not suitable for you.

Chapter 10 pulls everything together and can act as a guide to support you through the often overwhelming amount of information and options.

Our greatest wish is that the information contained in this book will help your menopause transition to be as smooth as possible and that you have the energy and vigour to really enjoy this period of your life.

Chapter 1

OVERVIEW AND THE EXPERIENCE OF THE MENOPAUSE

In this introductory chapter we'll outline factual information regarding the physiological changes that occur within the menopause and the common symptoms women experience during this time. Next, we will cover known risk factors for diseases associated with increasing age and menopause, such as osteoporosis and heart disease. The good news is that many risk factors for these conditions are modifiable and there is action you can take to reduce your risk, which we explain below. Finally we'll explore both positive and negative consequences of the menopausal transition and more general aspects of ageing. We believe that whilst it's helpful to be aware of the more unwelcome features of the menopause, it's also useful to consider research and women's personal experiences that demonstrate the advantages of the cessation of menstruation. Of course when you are symptomatic these benefits may feel distant, but there are strategies that can facilitate wellbeing and physical health at this time, which we will discuss later in this book.

Physiology of the menopause

The average age of natural menopause is 51. Although life expectancy has improved considerably, the average age of menopause has not changed since records began, which means that women now spend about one third of their lives past menopause.

Before 'official' menopause, which is when you have not had a period for 12 months, there is a transition period, called perimenopause, which can last anything from five to 10 years. This is when you may start to notice changes in your menstrual cycle with periods becoming very unpredictable, often more frequent and heavier, followed by the possibility of no periods at all for 60 days or more. It can take anything from five to eight years after your final period before hormone levels settle.[1]

Why does menopause happen?

At birth, women have over a million egg cells (oocytes). By the time a woman reaches her forties, there may be a few thousand left, and few or none postmenopause. It is the depletion of oocytes which eventually leads to the cessation of menstruation. This is where the word menopause comes from, derived from the Greek 'men', meaning month, and 'pausis', which simply means 'a pause' or 'cessation'. Because we are running out of eggs, the oestrogen signal from our ovaries to our brain becomes weak (as do other hormone-stimulating signals) and ultimately no progesterone is produced because progesterone during the reproductive years is produced as oestrogen peaks at ovulation, which is no longer happening.

The menstrual cycle

The menstrual cycle typically lasts 28 days, although it can range from 23–35 days. Bleeding lasts on average for five days, although this too can vary from one to eight days. You can skip this section if you are already familiar with the endocrine system and the functions of oestrogen and progesterone during the menstrual cycle.

Figure 1.1 shows the different stages of the menstrual cycle and the rise and fall of oestrogen and progesterone.

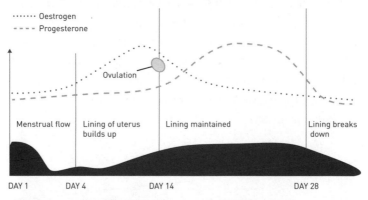

FIGURE 1.1 THE DIFFERENT STAGES OF THE MENSTRUAL CYCLE

From puberty, the ovaries release egg cells (ova). They also manufacture the sex hormones that influence the menstrual cycle and the development of female characteristics. Each ovary contains numerous cell clusters called follicles, in which egg cells develop. The growth of the follicle is initiated by a hormone called follicle-stimulating hormone (FSH), which also causes oestrogen to be secreted inside the developing follicle. Then another hormone called luteinising hormone (LH), kicks in, which stimulates further development of the follicle and secretion of oestrogen, and triggers ovulation mid-cycle. At ovulation, the follicle ruptures, releasing the mature egg into the fallopian tubes. The empty follicle develops into a small tissue mass, known as the corpus luteum, which secretes progesterone and oestrogen.

After ovulation, the corpus luteum produces progesterone, which acts on the womb lining and causes it to thicken in preparation for a fertilised egg to implant. This is known as the luteal phase of the menstrual cycle. If the egg is fertilised by a sperm and implants successfully into the womb, the corpus luteum continues to produce progesterone to maintain the pregnancy until the placenta develops fully. The placenta produces increasing amounts of progesterone until it is fully developed, when it then takes over the production of progesterone to continue to support the pregnancy. Rather than oestrogen and progesterone levels dipping, as they do at around day 25 of a 28-day cycle (which leads to menstruation), both hormone levels continue to rise, with progesterone levels actually becoming higher than oestrogen around this time.

What are hormones?

Some women have asked us what the word 'hormone' actually means. It comes from the Greek 'hormon', which means to 'set in motion' or to 'stimulate'. Hormones are chemicals, secreted into the bloodstream from various tissues and glands, such as the ovaries and the pancreas, that regulate body functions such as metabolism, growth and sexual reproduction. All the tissues and glands that produce hormones in different parts of the body are collectively known as the endocrine system.

The importance of cholesterol

Some people may find it surprising that all steroid hormones are made from cholesterol, which is actually a vital substance in your body. Cholesterol is converted by enzymes into pregnenolone, which is the 'master' hormone, as shown in Figure 1.2.

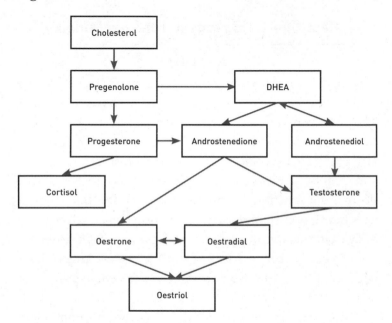

FIGURE 1.2 HOW HORMONES ARE CONVERTED FROM CHOLESTEROL IN THE BODY

What about 'bad' cholesterol?

When most people talk about cholesterol, they talk about 'good' (high-density lipoprotein, or HDL) and 'bad'(low-density lipoprotein, or LDL) – what they are actually referring to is the two 'transport carriers' (lipoproteins) that carry cholesterol in the blood. HDL reduces and recycles LDL, by transporting it to the liver where it can be reprocessed. LDL cholesterol is considered to be 'bad' cholesterol because it contributes to plaque, which is a thick, hard deposit that can clog arteries and make them less flexible. This condition is known as atherosclerosis. If a clot forms and blocks a narrowed artery, heart attack or stroke can result. LDL cholesterol is only 'bad' when it is oxidised (we'll explain more about how to prevent this happening in the next chapter).

Oestrogen and progesterone explained

Oestrogen

Oestrogen promotes development and maintenance of the female reproductive system and female characteristics. It also acts on many non-reproductive organs and systems in the body. Cells in the vagina, bladder, breasts, skin, bones, arteries, heart, liver, and brain all contain oestrogen receptors, and require oestrogen to stimulate these receptors for normal cell function (for example, to keep the skin smooth and moist, for proper bone formation, and to keep the body's internal thermostat operating properly). Oestrogen is not just *one* hormone – at least six different oestrogens have been identified, although only three are present in significant quantities:

Oestradiol (E2), or beta-oestradiol, is the most abundant form of oestrogen in non-pregnant women and is the primary oestrogen produced by your ovaries. Oestradiol is also the strongest oestrogen and the one you have most of during your reproductive years. This form of oestrogen is tested to determine blood levels of oestrogen and also the form of oestrogen in many different forms of hormone replacement therapy (HRT) (see Chapters 7 and 8).

Oestrone (E1) is produced when your liver converts oestradiol to oestrone. This is the form of oestrogen you have the most of in your postmenopause years (if you're not taking oestrogen replacement).

Oestriol (E3) is the weakest form of oestrogen and is highest during pregnancy as the placenta produces high amounts to protect the foetus. This form of oestrogen appears not to overstimulate breast and uterine tissues as the other forms of oestrogen do and is believed to be protective against breast cancer.

Progesterone

Progesterone is essential for the normal functioning of the reproductive system. This hormone acts together with oestrogen to prepare and then maintain the womb for implantation of a fertilised egg, and to prepare the mammary glands for milk secretion. After ovulation, the corpus luteum (which is the empty follicle from which the egg was released) produces progesterone, which causes the womb lining to thicken in preparation for a fertilised egg to implant. This is known as the luteal phase of the menstrual cycle. If an egg implants successfully into the womb, the corpus luteum continues to produce progesterone to maintain the pregnancy until the placenta develops fully. The placenta produces increasing amounts of progesterone until it is fully developed, when it then takes over the production of progesterone to continue to support the pregnancy.

Premature and early-onset menopause

Menopause may also be induced prematurely (before the age of 40) or early (before the age of 45) through medical interventions such as surgery (for example, removal of the ovaries, with or without hysterectomy), chemotherapy, or radiation. Some researchers have also linked early menopause with exposure to a group of chemicals, known as endocrine-disrupting chemicals, or EDCs (see box on page 20).

Sometimes you will see them referred to as xenoestrogens. In particular, perfluorochemicals (PFCs) have been associated with early menopause, as much as 3.8 years earlier in women with the highest levels.[2]

Endocrine-disrupting chemicals (EDCs)

Industrialisation has led to the production of thousands of chemicals used in the manufacturing of pharmaceuticals, pesticides, textiles, furniture, flame retardants, personal care and household cleaning products, and other common household items. EDCs are chemicals or combinations of chemicals that interfere with any aspect of human hormonal action. We will talk more about these in the next chapter and give you information on how to reduce your exposure.

Premature ovarian insufficiency

There is also a condition called premature ovarian insufficiency (POI), which is said to have occurred when menstruation ceases before the age of 40, although this is quite rare (approximately 1 per cent of women younger than 40, 0.1 per cent under 30 and 0.01 per cent under 20).[3]

If you are under 40 and have erratic periods, for which pregnancy has been excluded, you should have your hormone levels tested, including serum levels of FSH, oestradiol and thyroid hormones. If the FSH level is within the hormonal range, this should be re-tested before any diagnosis is made as levels can fluctuate. Although pregnancy in patients with POI is unlikely and rare, the condition is not necessarily permanent and spontaneous pregnancies have been reported to be 5–10 per cent.[4] Please see Chapter 8 for details of how POI can be managed with HRT.

What to expect during the transition phase (perimenopause)

What happens first are anovulatory cycles, which means cycles where no ovulation occurs. These become progressively more common, although you will not necessarily be aware of this. The first thing you are likely to notice is changes in your menstrual cycle such as irregularities, or increased blood flow. Eventually, the first part of your cycle (follicular phase) shortens, and the latter part of your cycle varies considerably from month to month (luteal phase). Research has shown that symptoms of menopause generally begin two to three years before the final menstrual period, peak during the first year after the final menstrual period, and then diminish. If three or more menstruations are missed within a 12 month period it is likely that the menopause transition will be completed within four years. There can be continued oestrogen production in the absence of progesterone leading to possible thickening of the womb lining. As a result, menstruation can become heavy, prolonged, and unpredictable with intermenstrual bleeding.

Common symptoms

Although some women do not experience any troublesome symptoms during the menopause, approximately 85 per cent of women have symptoms that vary in type and severity. A European survey of 4200 women, aged 45–59, revealed that they nearly all experienced one or more postmenopausal symptoms, with 63 per cent of them rating these symptoms as severe. The most frequently reported symptoms were:

▶ hot flushes (74 per cent)

▶ sleeplessness (58 per cent)

▶ mood changes (57 per cent)

▶ irritability (53 per cent)

▶ reduced sex drive (45 per cent).

Most women indicated that hot flushes was the symptom that most affected their lives and caused them to seek treatment, followed by sleeplessness and mood swings.[5] Women with mild or moderate symptoms may opt not to use any treatment or use a herbal/natural remedy (see Chapter 3) because of the risks associated with HRT, which we cover in detail (as well as the benefits) in Chapters 7 and 8.

Vasomotor symptoms

Hot flushes (or flashes)

Hot flushes are one of the most frequently reported and wearing symptoms that occur during perimenopause and menopause. Hot flushes help the body to dissipate heat and usually consist of face, chest, and neck sweating. Increased skin temperature and blood flow (due to widening of the veins and arteries) also occur, lasting around 1–5 minutes. Estimates of the average length of time women will experience hot flushes varies widely from a matter of months to a decade, with those that experience hot flushes early in their menopause more likely to have this symptom for longer.[6] Ethnicity and body weight appear to increase the likelihood of experiencing this symptom, and experiencing it for a greater length of time, with women from African origins and those defined as obese having greater risk. Anxiety also appears to play a part in the probability of hot flushes occurring and stress, alcohol and coffee have all been shown to be a trigger for this symptom. Not only are hot flushes distressing in themselves, they can also cause embarrassment and affect sleep quality.

Night sweats

When hot flushes occur whilst sleeping, they can produce intense perspiration that can cause women to wake, often needing a change of clothing and/or bedding as a result. Some women also have difficulty falling asleep again. This can be extremely distressing and can drain your energy and have other knock-on effects, such as constant fatigue, concentration and memory problems, depression, and low sex drive.

Urogenital symptoms

The term 'urogenital atrophy' refers to changes in the vagina and lower urinary tract which occur due to declining oestrogen levels in these tissues. Urinary incontinence, increased frequency and urinary tract infections may be an issue.

Vaginal dryness and pain

The term 'vaginal atrophy' is used to describe the changes in the vaginal walls that occur during the menopause. The change in hormone levels can cause the tissue lining the inside of the vagina (vaginal epithelium) to become thin, dry, and sometimes inflamed. These changes cause discomfort during intercourse and pelvic examinations.

Loss of libido

Not surprisingly, the vaginal changes and pain during intercourse (dyspareunia) mentioned above can lead to decreased libido. This is a common problem for both peri- and postmenopausal women. There are also psychological aspects at this time which we will cover later in this chapter.

Somatic symptoms

Headaches and migraines

For most people, a headache happens occasionally and can be quickly cured with something to eat or drink, a short rest, or a couple of painkillers. Only a few (around 5 per cent) are a sign that something is seriously wrong. Get medical advice urgently if your headache occurs suddenly and severely, especially after a blow to the head, if it has been present for some time, or if it's accompanied by a fever, rash, or feelings of drowsiness.

Migraines are much more than just a headache, which typically consist of a moderate-to-severe throbbing pain that is worse on one side of the head. This is usually accompanied by other symptoms, such as nausea, vomiting, and sensitivity to light and noise. They usually last four to 72 hours and may occur rarely or up to several times a week. Migraines can occur with or without an 'aura', which means you may experience other symptoms before a migraine begins such as yawning, seeing flashing lights and floating lines, or developing temporary peripheral blindness, numbness or tingling in the face or hands, distorted sense of smell, taste, or touch, and mental confusion or slurred speech. Although these symptoms can be frightening they are not normally the sign of a serious underlying condition. However, if you do have frequent migraines please consult your doctor who may want to refer you to a specialist, or headache and migraine clinic.

WHAT CAUSES MIGRAINES AND HOW
SHOULD THEY BE TREATED?

The causes of migraines are not fully understood, but researchers think that changes in levels of brain chemicals can cause inflammation, making blood vessels swell and press on nearby nerves. They're often connected to fluctuations in oestrogen, which could explain why around two-thirds of migraines are in women. Hormonal migraines may also be related to changes in the amount of a chemical called serotonin in the brain and some medications are designed to correct that imbalance. You are more likely to have migraines if they run in your family.

IDENTIFYING MIGRAINE TRIGGERS

Women who suffer from migraines usually become aware of 'triggers', such as bright or flashing lights, lack of food or sleep, a particular food or group of foods that they react to, stress, and/or changes in hormone levels. A good way to identify triggers and manage your migraines is to keep a diary of when they occur (see Chapter 6). This will help you to identify if your migraines or headaches have any relation to your hormone levels.

HORMONAL MIGRAINES

Every woman is different but you may find that migraines become less severe if they were linked to your menstrual cycle. However, you may get them for the first time or they may worsen around perimenopause because of new hormonal fluctuations. The good news is that hormonal migraines usually stop after menopause, when hormone levels are consistently low. If your migraines are hormonal, the main goal of your treatment should be to stabilise your oestrogen levels (HRT may be an option for you; see Chapters 7 and 8) and you should discuss this with your doctor.

Treatments without medication include relaxation techniques, changes in diet (Chapters 2 and 3), stress reduction, acupuncture, and regular sleep/wake schedules (Chapters 4, 5, and 6). Medications, such as magnesium or aspirin, (triptans and nonsteroidal anti-inflammatory drugs) can prevent migraines from occurring or stop a migraine that has already begun.

Palpitations

Heart palpitations are heartbeats that suddenly become more noticeable, such as fluttering or beating irregularly, often for just a few seconds or minutes. Palpitations can sometimes be the result of hormonal changes around the time of the menopause and are usually temporary and not a cause for concern. However, if you start to experience palpitations more often, or if they get worse or occur with other symptoms such as dizziness, fatigue, shortness of breath, or tightness in your chest, you should see your GP as they may be a sign of a heart rhythm problem (arrhythmia). Your GP can carry out tests to assess your heart rate and rhythm and determine if treatment is necessary.

Heart palpitations may be triggered by a surge of adrenaline, eating rich, spicy foods, and/or consuming too much caffeine or alcohol. Other underlying causes include an overactive thyroid, low blood sugar, anaemia, low blood pressure, fever, and dehydration.

Psychological symptoms

We cover the psychological aspects of menopause later in this chapter and throughout the book. Many women ask, 'is it me or is it my hormones and how do I know the difference?' Clearly psychology affects physiology and vice versa – in fact, there are areas of research dedicated to this mind–brain–body interface (see Chapter 5).

Depression

Depressive symptoms can range from a depressed mood to clinical depression. A depressed mood (which occurs in approximately one-third of postmenopausal women) may not require treatment, but if clinical depression is suspected, assessment and treatment are recommended. Women suffering from depression (which is associated with a chemical imbalance in the brain) report symptoms of prolonged tiredness, loss of interest in normal activities, weight gain/loss, sadness, or irritability. Treatments can include talk therapy and herbal remedies such as St John's wort for mild to moderate depression (Chapter 3), and prescription medications and/or talk therapy if more severe.

Anxiety

Symptoms of anxiety may include tension, nervousness, panic, and worry. Physical and psychological changes as well as other midlife stressors can result in increased anxiety. Sometimes anxiety can lead to panic attacks, causing shortness of breath, chest pain, sweating, dizziness, and heart palpitations. Although they can be frightening and intense, they aren't usually dangerous. Treatments include relaxation or stress reduction techniques, counselling or psychotherapy, and/or prescription drugs.

Insomnia and sleep disturbances

Sleep disturbances occur in more than 40 per cent of menopausal women. Insomnia can include lengthy times to fall asleep, inability to sleep through the night, or inability to resume sleep when waking prematurely. If you think you might suffer from sleep apnoea, where symptoms range from slight airflow reductions causing snoring to periodic cessation of breathing, you should see your doctor.

When should I seek medical help?

As we've previously mentioned, some symptoms of menopause, such as heart palpitations and fatigue, can be a sign of other health issues. For example, thyroid disorders are common in women and can be diagnosed with a simple blood test. It is important to see your doctor if you are unsure so that s/he can assess your symptoms and/or carry out tests to determine the root cause. Some women are reluctant to ask for help from their doctors as they may be too embarrassed or think they are wasting their time. Some women have even been 'fobbed off' in the past and told it's their age and are reluctant to return. If you are not happy with your current doctor, you are entitled to ask to see a different one who can be sympathetic to your needs. It may be worthwhile to ask which doctor in your local surgery has specific expertise in women's health and then ask to be seen by him or her. It's very important that you don't try to diagnose and treat yourself but rather receive the support and care from your doctor and/or specialists or private therapists such as psychologists (Chapter 4) or Complementary and Alternative Medicine (CAM) practitioners (Chapter 5).

Associated health issues

There are long-term effects of declining hormone levels that are important for a woman to consider. As previously mentioned, oestrogen receptors are not just found in the ovaries and breasts, they are also found in the heart, blood vessels, bones, bladder, skin, even your brain. So there are long-term health risks associated with the menopause, such as an increased risk of heart attack, stroke, breast cancer, and osteoporosis. But these health problems are not foregone conclusions by any means. Below we cover the risk factors for these conditions, together with action you can take to minimise your risk. It goes without saying that factors such as poor diet, high alcohol consumption, smoking, and sedentary lifestyle/lack of exercise all increase your risk of many illnesses so we will not repeat them continuously. So, assume these are all risk factors and also consider the additional risk factors in each section.

Family history and genetics

Scientists have been aware for some time that the genes we inherit from our parents may partly determine whether we will develop specific diseases, including osteoporosis, heart disease, dementia, and cancer. Some genes may not actually cause the illness, but may affect your risk. For example, a number of genes have been identified that do not directly cause dementia but are thought to affect a person's risk of developing the disease, such as a gene called apolipoprotein E. This gene has been shown to play a part in the development of heart disease, Alzheimer's disease, and vascular dementia. It is also possible to inherit genes that can directly cause dementia, although these are much rarer than the risk genes. For example, there are some families in which there is a very clear inheritance of dementia from one generation to the next. Dementia-causing diseases that are hereditary include Huntington's disease and familial Alzheimer's disease (a very rare form of Alzheimer's with onset before the age of 60). In these cases what is being passed on from parent to child are specific genes that directly cause dementia. Although researchers have made some important advances in recent years, the role of genetics is still not fully understood and therefore beyond the scope of this book.

Osteoporosis

Bone is a living tissue. Throughout our lives, bones are continually being broken down and rebuilt to facilitate growth and repair. Bones have two types of cells, bone-building cells (called osteoblasts) and bone-clearing cells (called osteoclasts). In young people, the rate of bone formation exceeds the rate at which bone is broken down, or resorbed, by the body. This process begins to change in early adulthood, with bone being cleared faster than it is being formed, causing the bones to become weaker and lighter. Peak bone mass, which is the time when bones reach their maximum density and strength, occurs in women around the ages of 25–30. From then until menopause, there are minimal changes in total bone mass, unless any of the risk factors below apply. However, in the first few years after menopause, most women experience rapid bone loss, which then slows but continues throughout the postmenopausal years. This loss of bone mass can lead to osteoporosis, which is a bone-weakening disorder.

There are a number of additional risk factors that can increase your likelihood of developing osteoporosis including:

▶ late menses/early menopause (less exposure to oestrogen during your lifetime)

▶ surgery to remove both ovaries before natural menopause

▶ insufficient calcium throughout life

▶ gaps in menstruation (due to low body weight or excessive exercise)

▶ prolonged use of steroid medication

▶ eating disorders

▶ lack of weight-bearing exercise, such as walking, jogging, tennis

▶ being thin or having a low body weight.

The good news

There is a lot you can do to prevent and treat osteoporosis, which we cover throughout this book. Oestrogen and progesterone are vital to the bone-building process, which is why menopausal women are particularly susceptible as oestrogen and progesterone levels decline. HRT is covered in Chapters 7 and 8. There are many other factors involved in this process such as vitamins and minerals, covered in Chapter 3, and exercise (especially weight-bearing), covered in Chapter 6. Medical management is covered in Chapter 9.

Cardiovascular issues

Cardiovascular disease (CVD) is the leading cause of death for women, accounting for approximately 45 per cent of mortality. Before the menopause, women have a much lower risk of heart attack and stroke than men, although this risk becomes the same as men within ten years after the menopause. A great deal of research has been devoted to determine if oestrogen is protective for the heart and this is covered in Chapters 7 and 8.

The additional risk factors for CVD are:

▶ high blood pressure

▶ high cholesterol

▶ blood that clots easily

▶ being overweight

▶ too much stress

▶ depression.

The good news

There is a lot you can do to protect your heart and circulation. By staying active, eating well, not smoking, and keeping your stress levels to a minimum, the risk of CVD can be reduced Stress in life is inevitable so it is vital to find a way to minimise the effects that stress has on your body (see Chapter 6).

Cognitive function

It is important to remember that forgetfulness is common at any age. Many perimenopausal women report difficulty concentrating or short-term memory problems. These are common complaints by midlife women but some women may worry that they have early symptoms of Alzheimer's disease, which is rarely the case.

A study measured cognitive performance in a group of women going through the menopause transition and found that the natural menopause transition was not associated with memory decline. Although the perimenopausal women were not able to learn as well as they had during premenopause, improvement returned to premenopausal levels in postmenopause, suggesting that cognitive difficulties during the menopause transition may be only temporary.

The risk factors for cognitive difficulties such as problems with memory and attention are as follows:

▶ Increasing age – dementia is rare before 65 years of age (earlier forms tend to be very different from late-onset) and is estimated to affect one in 14 people over the age of 65 and one in six over the age of 80. This increased risk may be due to factors associated with ageing, such as changes to DNA and the weakening of the body's natural repair systems.

▶ Women are slightly more likely to develop Alzheimer's disease than men. One factor that has been suggested in the development of Alzheimer's disease is a lack of oestrogen in women after the menopause (see Chapter 7).

▶ Having a close relative (parent or sibling) with the disease may increase the risk.

▶ Medical history – conditions that affect the heart, arteries, or blood circulation all significantly affect a person's chances of developing dementia, particularly vascular dementia. These conditions include diabetes, and midlife high blood pressure, high blood cholesterol levels, and obesity. Stroke is a major risk factor for dementia.

▶ Depression – this may be a risk factor for dementia, or an early symptom of the disease.

▶ Severe or repeated head injuries may increase the risk of developing cognitive difficulties.

▶ Alcohol – drinking above recommended levels significantly increases the risk of Alzheimer's and vascular dementia. However, research suggests that light-to-moderate amounts of alcohol may protect the brain against dementia and keep the heart and vascular system healthy. People who regularly drink excessive amounts of alcohol over a long period of time are at risk of developing Korsakoff's syndrome and other alcohol-related dementias.

The good news

Studies suggest that remaining physically, socially, and mentally active may help prevent memory loss and reduce your risks of developing dementia. Check if you are a healthy weight for your height and change your lifestyle to incorporate regular exercise in the long term (aim to be physically active for at least 30 minutes, five times a week). The exercise you do should be of moderate intensity, which means that you should be working hard enough to raise your heart rate and break a sweat. Examples include cycling or taking a brisk walk.

Research also suggests that people who take part in mental activities (such as reading, learning, and doing puzzles) are less likely to develop dementia compared with those who do not. It is thought that mental activity increases the brain's ability to cope with, and compensate for, damage and that a person who often takes part in these activities will be able to tolerate a greater level of damage before symptoms of dementia are detected.

If you are over 40, or have a history of dementia or cardiovascular problems in your family, you should get regular blood pressure and cholesterol checks to ensure these are within recommended levels. Managing your cholesterol by eating a balanced diet that avoids saturated fats will also help. It is also important to keep diabetes under control and seek early treatment for depression.

If you smoke, please consult your doctor for help to stop. This will be of huge benefit to your health in a number of ways as well as reducing your risk of dementia. Your doctor can provide help and advice about quitting, and can refer you to a support service if necessary.

Breast cancer

Breast cancer is the most common cancer in the UK. The lifetime risk of being diagnosed with breast cancer is one in eight for women in the UK and about 12,000 women in the UK die of breast cancer every year. However, survival rates have been improving over the years and now about three of four women diagnosed with breast cancer are alive 10 years later.

In Europe, more than 464,000 new cases of breast cancer were estimated to have been diagnosed in 2012. The UK incidence rate is sixth highest in Europe. Worldwide, it is estimated that more than 1.68 million women were diagnosed with breast cancer in 2012, with incidence rates varying across the world.

The additional risk factors for developing breast cancer are:

▶ Increasing age – about four out of five cases of breast cancer are found in women over 50 years old.

▶ Having a close relative (mother, sister or grandmother) who has had breast cancer. (Although not all women with breast cancer have a family history of the disease and having a family history does not mean you will inevitably develop breast cancer. However, you should let your doctor know if any of your close relatives have been diagnosed with it so that you can be monitored.)

▶ Late menopause (after age 55).

▶ Starting menstruation early in life (before age 12).

▶ Having a first child after age 30.

▶ Never having children.

▶ Being overweight.

▶ Not breastfeeding.

The good news

Research shows that up to 40 per cent of cancers are preventable through diet and lifestyle changes. This is covered in more detail in the next chapter.

Checking your breasts and Breast Screening Programmes

If you get to know how your breasts normally look and feel, you will be more likely to notice any changes that could be signs of breast cancer. Being diagnosed and treated at an early stage increases your chances of survival so you should check your breasts on a regular basis (at least once a month). It is very important to see your doctor if you notice any changes in your breast, such as:

▶ a lump or thickening that you can see or feel

▶ any changes in the skin, such as dimpling of the skin

▶ any changes in the nipple, such as change of shape, rash, or any blood or other fluid coming from the nipple

▶ pain or discomfort in the breast or armpit

▶ a swelling or lump in the armpit.

Breast screening in the UK

All women aged 50–70 are invited for screening (mammogram) every three years. A mammogram is an x-ray, and therefore not without risks. To help keep your breast still and get a clear picture a plastic plate is lowered onto your breast to flatten it, which can be uncomfortable and some women find it quite painful. To help you decide, we have summarised below the positives and negatives of screening, as detailed in the National Health Service (NHS) Breast Screening leaflet:

POSITIVES

▶ Screening saves about one life from breast cancer for every 200 women who are screened. This adds up to about 1300 lives saved from breast cancer each year in the UK.

▶ 96 out of every 100 women screened will show no sign of cancer.

▶ About four in every 100 will be asked to go back for more tests, such as breast examination, ultrasound scan, or biopsy.

▶ Of these four women, one will be found to have cancer.

▶ About one in five women diagnosed with breast cancer will have non-invasive cancer, which means that the cancer cells are contained within the milk ducts (tubes) and have not spread further. This is also called ductal carcinoma in situ (DCIS). In some women, the cancer cells stay inside the ducts, although in others they can grow into the surrounding breast in the future. Doctors can't always tell whether a non-invasive breast cancer will grow into the surrounding breast or not, or whether a breast cancer will go on to be life-threatening, so they offer treatment to all women with breast cancer. This means that some women will be offered treatment that they do not need. About four in five women will have invasive cancer, which means that the cancer has grown out of the milk ducts and into the surrounding breast. Most invasive breast cancers will spread to other parts of the body if left untreated.

NEGATIVES

▶ The main risk is that screening can find cancers that would never have caused harm. Some women will be diagnosed and treated unnecessarily. About three in every 200 women screened every three years from the age of 50 to 70 are diagnosed with a cancer that would never have been found without screening and would never have become life-threatening. This adds up to about 4000 women each year in the UK who are offered treatment they did not need.

▶ Most women who receive an abnormal screening result are found not to have breast cancer. However, these women have still experienced unnecessary worry and distress, which can affect their quality of life.

▶ Rarely, cancers can be missed – most are picked up but breast cancer is missed in about one in 2500 women screened.

▶ Having mammograms every three years for 20 years very slightly increases the chance of getting cancer over a woman's lifetime (although x-rays can rarely cause cancer).

Overall, for every one woman who has her life saved from breast cancer, about three women are diagnosed with a cancer that would never have been life-threatening. Therefore, it is *your* choice whether you decide to have breast screening.

Type 2 diabetes

Since 1996, the number of people with diabetes in the UK has risen from 1.4 million to 3.2 million (6 per cent of the population). Diabetes prevalence in the UK is estimated to rise to five million by 2025. It is estimated that 382 million people worldwide are living with diabetes, which is estimated to be 8.5 per cent of the world's population.

Does menopause increase diabetes risk? That hasn't been an easy question for researchers to answer. It's hard to separate the effects of menopause from the effects of age and weight. Going through the menopause *per se* does not increase your risk for diabetes. However, changes in the levels of oestrogen and progesterone can lead to unexpected fluctuations in your blood sugars, making it harder to prevent diabetes and keep it well controlled. Putting on weight is a common issue for some women who go through menopause and after menopause, and can increase the need for insulin or oral diabetes medication. Diabetes raises the risk of urinary and vaginal infections, and this risk increases further during and after menopause as less oestrogen in the body makes for even more ideal conditions in the urinary tract/vagina for bacteria and yeast to thrive in. Sleep problems, perhaps caused by hot flushes and night sweats, can cause sleepless nights which, in turn, can have a negative impact on blood glucose control.

The additional risk factors for developing Type 2 diabetes are:

▶ being overweight or having a high Body Mass Index (BMI)

▶ carrying excess weight around your waist. A large waist is considered more than 80cm/31.5 inches in women; 94cm/37 inches in men; or 89cm/35 inches in South Asian men

▶ being from an African-Caribbean, Black African, Chinese or South Asian background and over 25

▶ being from another ethnic background and over 40

▶ having a parent, brother, or sister with diabetes

▶ having ever had high blood pressure, a heart attack, or a stroke

▶ a history of polycystic ovaries, gestational diabetes, or if you have given birth to a baby over 10 pounds/4.5kg

▶ suffering from schizophrenia, bipolar illness or depression, or taking anti-psychotic medication.

The good news

There are many things you can do to reduce your risk, such as achieving and maintaining a healthy body weight, being physically active (at least 30 minutes of regular, moderate-intensity activity on most days), and eating a healthy balanced diet (see Chapter 2). Exercise and managing stress levels can both help to stabilise blood sugar levels (see Chapter 6).

Impact on life

Associated with the physiological alternations outlined above, there are physical changes and emotional and social adjustments that occur during the menopause. For some women, the timing of menopause may coincide with other stresses like relationship issues, divorce or widowhood, struggles with adolescents, return of grown children to the home, being childless, concerns about ageing parents and caregiving responsibilities, as well as career and education issues. Although the health issues linked to hormonal fluctuations may appear wholly negative, this is not to say that all the experiences women have at this time are undesirable. Seeing the end of menstruation, lessened child-rearing responsibilities, and growth in personal confidence can all be beneficial life changes. However, this is not to deny that the menopausal transition can be distressing; hence we will first discuss some of the challenging experiences that women sometimes face during this period.

Bodily change

With the decline in reproductive hormones, physical appearance can subtly, or dramatically, change. Even if some women do not have menopausal symptoms and welcome the transition, bodily alterations can taint the experience.

This is unsurprising when confronted with thinning hair, dry skin, weight gain, and loss of breast fullness. Our intrinsic views of ourselves can be challenged as our external features morph and our body image is re-evaluated. But there are ways to help with this adjustment that will be presented in Chapter 6.

Body image

The impact of the menopause on women's views of their bodies is complex.[7] Ratings of body image don't simply slide as women enter into the perimenopause and menopause, even if physical appearance alters. Body image is not only an important concept for women themselves in their daily life, but also for partners and medical professionals to be aware of. Beliefs surrounding body image can affect psychological wellbeing and similarly depression and anxiety can influence self-perceptions. Therefore finding ways to boost body confidence can be a key to maintaining both emotional and physical health not only during the menopause, but throughout life (see Chapter 6).

Australian psychologist and researcher Amanda Deeks noted the intricate relationship between emotional wellbeing and body image in 2003.[8] Dr Deeks emphasised the importance of understanding the context of women when thinking about symptoms as there are numerous aspects of our culture and environment that worsen symptoms. For instance, trying to pertain to a cultural norm of what a women should look like and how one should behave can be exhausting and quite frankly, futile. However, the positive counter view to this is that these issues can be tackled in each woman's life, resulting in improved menopausal and psychological symptoms.

Age, not stage

Further research by Dr Deeks, along with colleague Marita McCabe, looked at differences in body image between groups of premenopausal, menopausal and postmenopausal women. Although there was a general trend for women to feel less attractive as they got older, the stage of menopause they were at did not affect their body image ratings. In other words, although views of physical appearance did diminish with increasing years, the menopause in itself did not lead women to feel less attractive.[9] Even though this might seem little comfort, there was an even more notable finding in this study: when taking into account women's perceptions of their shape and their views on the society's ideal body shape, the researchers observed that the assumed societal 'ideal' was unrealistically small for most women. This means that even if the women were content with their body shape, they believed society would judge them as 'not ideal' which could lead to feelings of dissatisfaction. So again, finding ways to feel comfortable and confident in your own skin may be an important aspect to tackle, rather than, or in addition to, individual symptoms *per se*.

Becoming invisible

Feeling good about ourselves can be difficult though, especially if there is a sense of becoming 'invisible'. In a study carried out within the Division of Social and Developmental Psychology at the University of Cambridge, researchers found that many women felt they had suddenly become invisible in society once their physical appearance started to change.[10] A diminishing sense of validation and worth as an individual was cited by the interviewees, even though they still felt worthy of attention. It should be noted however that the heterosexual women in this study most commonly expressed this concern in relation to men. Furthermore, women who judged themselves on physical characteristics, rather than competencies and general health, appeared to find this more problematic, whereas those who acknowledged some of the positive aspects of the menopause (see below) retained their feeling of visibility and value.

Not all bad...

To this point we've discussed mainly negative aspects of the menopause and ageing but there are positives too. Dr Lotte Hvas, a Danish GP with a keen interest in patient-centred medicine (who takes the approach that each patient should be considered as a unique individual, with her own beliefs, values, and experiences), has focused her research not just on the undesirable aspects of the menopause but also looked at the advantages of this transition:

> Being a female general practitioner, aged in the mid-forties, my curiosity has been triggered by the experiences from my work. It is my impression that women have a more differentiated and many facetted experience of menopause than is described in medical literature or advertisements. In fact the myth about the suffering, oestrogen-depleted menopausal women does not seem to be in agreement with the women I often see in general practice as well-being, good looking, healthy women often in the prime of life, even if some of the women, of course, do have symptoms.[11]

This reflects our own experience and observations; therefore this final portion of this chapter is dedicated to exploring the improvements in life women can enjoy during and after the menopause.

Relief from menstruation

One positive aspect of the menopause that Dr Hvas has noted in her work is the relief from menstruation and its associated difficulties.[12,13] On a completely practical note, women who were surveyed and interviewed in Dr Hvas' studies mentioned that the cessation of periods meant no longer needing to purchase, carry, and use tampons and sanitary towels. Not having to worry about menstruation during holidays and no longer considering contraception were also practical benefits stated. Menstrual periods in themselves can cause a raft of symptoms including premenstrual syndrome (PMS), migraines, spotting and irregular bleeding, and severe cramps, so the absence of these symptoms can offer respite. Indeed, some women in Dr Hvas' questionnaire study said that previous bleeding irregularities caused a great deal of worry.[14] The survey respondents were also pleased to have seen an end to oedema (water retention), sore breasts, and monthly bouts of depression. Hence, although for a number of women the menopause can initiate unpleasant symptoms, for others is can close a chapter of bothersome and intrusive reoccurring symptoms.

Improved sex life

Contrary to the view that experiencing the menopause marks the termination of a fulfilling and enjoyable sex life, Dr Hvas and other commentators have found that the menopause can mark the beginning of a phase of sexual liberation.[15,16] For many women, the ease at which they feel with their partners following numerous years together can give rise to better sex lives; the fears, insecurities, and doubts associated with budding relationships are no longer present. This, in addition to the freedom from contraceptive concerns, can mark a new and exciting level of intimacy in sexual relationships.

Sense of attractiveness

When exploring the research on body image and the menopause, it appears that a sense of attractiveness can play a major part not only in emotional wellbeing but also somatic types of symptoms. An Austrian study that controlled for hormone levels found that women who were more satisfied with their physical appearance reported less menopausal symptoms.[17] There was also a link between self-esteem and symptom frequency, with women who had higher ratings of self-esteem experiencing less symptoms overall. Because this piece of research took into account the women's hormone levels, these differences in symptoms could not be explained by reductions in sex hormones, i.e. feeling good about oneself actually made experiencing menopausal symptoms less likely.

Perceived attractiveness can also help with maintaining a good sex life. In a study looking at current sexual satisfaction in 307 heterosexual women, those who viewed themselves as more attractive now than when they were younger desired and had sex more often, experienced better orgasms, and took more pleasure in sex overall.[18] The researchers also found that although perceived attractiveness did not differ between those who were experiencing the menopause and women who were not, women who thought they were less attractive than they once were saw a decline in their sexual activity. This study shows yet again the importance of self-perception and our thoughts and feelings when it comes to the impact of the menopause, which is an area we will talk about further in Chapter 6.

Increased confidence

In addition to an augmented sexual life and a heightened sense of freedom in menopausal women, a new sense of confidence and ability to be outspoken has been documented.

This might simply be a product of age and the accumulation of experience, rather than the menopause *per se*, but it is worth noting when considering the positive aspects of the menopause. Aforementioned researchers from the University of Cambridge reported that women felt more able to be open and speak their mind.[19] This finding was mirrored by Dr Hvas' work in Denmark, where the interviewees said that no longer felt restrained by the views of others and could now be more assertive and make personal demands that they could not previously.[20] Women at this stage of life have said that they felt stronger, more in contact with their feelings, and had fewer inhibitions.[21]

More freedom

There has been a great deal of research and commentary on the 'empty nest syndrome', i.e. the feeling of loss and sense of anxiety when children leave home. This may of course be compounded by the inability to have more children; however there are advantages of having adult children. There can be a feeling of freedom in being able to concentrate on personal needs once adult children fly the nest. The freedom brought about by no longer needing to care for children can be significant and women can begin to prioritise themselves.[22] Visits from offspring can be enjoyed but then the space, both actual and emotional, of having grown-up children who live separately can be savoured. This is in sharp contrast to the out-dated cultural view that a women's worth is based on her role in the family unit and the doom sometimes portrayed in terms of 'an empty nest'. The mark of the menopause and cessation of child bearing and rearing years can bring a fresh start where women can pursue their own interests and goals.[23,24] Of course for women without children this would not be an added benefit, but the practical advantages of no longer having menstrual periods, not needing to worry about contraception, possible heightened sex life, and increased confidence are benefits that all women can enjoy.

Chapter 1 summary

In this first chapter we have covered some quite technical physiological and medical information regarding the menopause. This may seem a little overwhelming and it's fine to feel like this when presented with information that can at first appear to be quite negative. However, the important point about giving you information regarding symptoms and possible associated health issues is so you can take positive steps in order to protect and improve your health. If you are struggling with menopausal symptoms or worried about conditions such as osteoporosis or breast cancer, the remainder of this book is dedicated to ways in which you can manage symptoms and reduce your chance of developing any of the health issues we've listed above. As mentioned, there are also many beneficial aspects of this time of life that can be enjoyed such as increased freedoms and relief from the monthly hassles of menstruation.

Chapter 2

BASIC PRINCIPLES FOR HORMONAL HEALTH

In the last chapter, we talked about long-term health issues associated with the menopause and outlined the main risk factors. The four most important lifestyle factors – smoking, diet, alcohol and bodyweight (all within our control) – accounted for 34 per cent of the cancers occurring in 2010.[25] We are continually asked, 'what is the most effective diet for weight-loss?', 'should I eat meat?', 'what about alcohol?' Everywhere you look there is information about the latest fad diet, or the latest 'cause' of cancer, and conflicting information about what you should, and shouldn't, eat. Life shouldn't be about giving up things you love – it should be about being responsible and aware of what you eat. In reality, everything in excess is harmful (even water) so moderation is key. Alcohol, red meat, and bacon, for example, are only harmful if consumed in excess – not if consumed as part of a healthy balanced diet.

Although this book isn't about cancer, it is probably one of the most feared diseases in our modern world. Breast cancer, for example, is the most common cancer in the UK and about four out of five cases of breast cancer are found in women over 50 years old. Many believe that there is little we can do about it – it is 'in our genes' or the 'luck of the draw' whether we get it or not. However, studies involving twins have really shed light on how much our lifestyle choices can affect our chances of contracting cancer. One study of 45,000 pairs of twins, published in the *New England Journal of Medicine* showed that up to 85 per cent of cancers could have been prevented, i.e. only 15 per cent were genetic. The researchers looked at non-shared environmental factors between the twins and estimated that choices such as diet, smoking, and exercise, accounted for 58 to 82 per cent of the cancers studied.[26]

Every ten years, the World Cancer Research Fund (WCRF) publishes a report based on an analysis of studies from around the world.[27] They pared down around half a million studies to the best 7000, and the results were then analysed by a panel of twenty-one leading scientists for their recommendations. They looked at 17 different types of cancer and a wide range of factors, mostly dietary, that can affect risk of developing the disease.

So, in this chapter, we will summarise the top ten WCRF recommendations as we believe that these are good advice for us all and basic principles for health that apply whatever your age and circumstances. We will also talk about other dietary measures you can take to improve your hormonal health and reduce your likelihood of long-term health issues associated with the menopause. Herbs and dietary supplements specifically for the menopause will be covered in the next chapter.

WCRF recommendations

The ten WCRF recommendations in 2007 were:

1. *Be as lean as possible within the normal range of body weight and avoid weight gain throughout adulthood:* A healthy weight is defined as having a body mass index (BMI) below 25. To find out your BMI, you can use an online calculator (see Useful Addresses/Websites), or ask your doctor to calculate it for you. Putting on weight during menopause can increase your breast cancer risk, even if you are within the healthy range. The WCRF experts found that at least six cancers – of the oesophagus, pancreas, bowel, breast postmenopause, kidney, and endometrium (womb lining) – were linked to obesity, and that the risks were increased by even quite modest weight gains.

2. *Be physically active as part of everyday life* (see Chapter 6).

3. *Limit consumption of energy-dense foods, and avoid sugary drinks* (see page 54).

4. *Eat mostly foods of plant origin.*

5. *Limit intake of red meat and avoid processed meat:* The report suggests moderation in the consumption of red meat, suggesting a limit of 500g (18oz) a week with very little, if any, being processed. Interestingly, their 'public health goal' is even lower at 300g (11oz) a week. This equates to a 150g (5.5oz) serving (roughly the size of your palm), twice a week. A total avoidance of processed meats is recommended because of convincing evidence that eating processed meat increases the risk of colon cancer. Processed meats include ham, bacon, salami or any other meat preserved by smoking,

curing, or salting. If you do consume red or processed meat, make sure you buy organic and/or free range wherever possible. Balance your weekly menus to include fish and organic poultry, and maybe consider going meat-free for one or two days of the week.

6. *Limit alcoholic drinks* (see page 60).

7. *Limit consumption of salt, and avoid mouldy cereals or pulses:* Adults should eat less than six grams of salt (2.5g of sodium) each day – that's about one teaspoon. This includes the salt that's contained within foods, as well as the salt you add to your food. Eating too much salt can raise blood pressure, which in turn increases your risk of developing heart disease.

8. *Aim to meet nutritional needs through diet alone:* Supplements must not take the place of a healthy diet and there is some evidence that certain supplements at high doses could have adverse effects. However, dietary supplements are valuable in some situations, such as stress, ill health, or dietary inadequacy. In our modern world, the foods we consume are less nutrient dense than the foods that our ancestors would have consumed. Foods can be depleted of nutrients due to modern farming methods; and extra nutrients are required to detoxify the many chemicals we are exposed to daily, such as endocrine disrupting chemicals (EDCs, see page 64). Most multivitamin and mineral combinations contain nutrients at safe levels and in the right combinations, and so a multi, together with extra vitamin C and essential fats, are considered as the 'basics' by many health experts. Please note we do not recommend taking high levels of individual nutrients unless advised by a health professional.

9. *If a new mother, breastfeed your baby.*

10. *Cancer survivors should follow the recommendations for cancer prevention.*

Interestingly, the WCRF report does not contain a recommendation about essential fatty acids, or EFAs, which are a vitally important component of any diet.

What are essential fatty acids (EFAs)?

There are two types of EFAs (also called polyunsaturated fatty acids, or PUFAs):

▶ omega-3

▶ omega-6.

Both have anti-inflammatory effects in the body. Most of us consume enough omega-6s in our diets, although it is possible to become deficient in omega-3s.

Omega-3s:

▶ reduce the risk of cardiovascular disease

▶ may reduce depression

▶ could slow cognitive decline.

Ensure you include sources of omega-3 fatty acids in your diet every day. Good sources include fish, especially fatty fish, such as mackerel, salmon, and sardines. Aim for two to three servings each week (as a guide: 80g oily or 150g white fish). If you don't eat fish, plant-based sources include nuts, seeds, seaweed, and soy.

What about saturated fat?

Too much saturated fat can cause narrowing of the arteries, making heart attack or stroke more likely. Heart attacks, stroke, and vascular disease increase a person's risk of developing vascular dementia. Limit saturated fat by choosing lean cuts of meat, trimming off any excess fat, and avoiding the skin on poultry and fish. Select extra lean mince or use a vegetarian alternative, such as soya mince.

The Ketogenic diet

Whilst we are on the subject of fats, we should mention the Ketogenic diet, which was originally developed for epilepsy but has been promoted in recent years as a diet for weight loss. This is a diet where carbohydrates are reduced and fats are increased so that the fat to carbohydrate ratio is 4:1, and protein is regulated so that around 90 per cent of calories are derived from fat. The theory behind this is that this way of eating forces the body to use ketone bodies as the predominant energy source, instead of glucose. Ketone bodies are molecules produced by the liver from fatty acids during periods of low food intake or carbohydrate restriction for cells of the body to use as energy. This diet should only be done under strict supervision by a health professional as it can have negative effects on the body, such as raised cholesterol and triglyceride levels, which are risk factors for heart attack and strokes.

Why is sugar so bad for us?

The most obvious reason to limit sugar in your diet is to keep your weight stable and avoid obesity. It is also important to keep your blood sugar level as stable as possible throughout the day for a number of reasons. First, you will feel better. Second, fluctuating blood sugar causes the body to store excess energy as fat and, as well as causing you to gain weight, in the long term this can lead to not only a lack of energy, but also an increased risk of diabetes and heart disease.

Certain types of carbohydrates increase glucose and insulin levels to a greater extent than others. High levels of insulin (hyperinsulinemia) can lead to a condition called insulin resistance (IR), which is a risk factor for diabetes. Hyperinsulinemia may in turn raise levels of proteins called insulin-like growth factors. High levels of insulin and insulin-like growth factor-I (IGF-I) are associated with an increased risk of breast cancer in several studies.[28]

What is energy density?

Because recommendation 3 of the WCRF report is 'Limit consumption of energy-dense foods, and avoid sugary drinks', we will give you some examples of how to do this.

'Energy density' is the amount of energy (or calories) per gram of food. Consuming high amounts of energy-dense foods can lead to excess weight or obesity, and increased risk of heart disease, osteoporosis, and cancer. It is very easy to calculate the energy density of foods, by dividing the number of calories by the weight (in grams). Studies have shown that people tend to consume about the same weight of food each day, but not necessarily the same amount of calories. Because lower energy-dense foods provide less energy per gram of food, you can eat more of them without consuming too many calories. So, although you may be eating the same weight of foods throughout the day, you will be consuming fewer calories, which will help you lose weight without feeling hungry.

Although it is better to eat mostly foods that are very low, low or medium in energy density, you can still consume higher energy-dense foods but just include them in smaller amounts. Here are some top tips for creating a lower energy-dense diet:

▶ Low energy dense foods (less than 1.5 calories/gram) should make up most of what we eat and include foods with a high water content, such as soups and stews, foods like pasta and rice that absorb water during cooking, and foods that are naturally high in water, such as fruit and vegetables. You can also add more liquids to dishes to help bulk them up without adding extra calories, such as adding an extra tin of tomatoes to a chilli or pasta sauce.

▶ Foods that are high in fibre (such as beans, and wholegrain rice, breads, pastas, and cereals), and lower fat foods (such as yogurts) also tend to have a lower energy density. Brown or wholegrain varieties of bread, rice, pasta, and breakfast cereals contain more fibre, which will help you feel fuller for longer.

▶ Bulk up meals by adding extra pulses, such as beans, peas, and lentils, which are high in fibre and protein, and filling, but low in calories. You could also add some extra rice or pasta to soups or salads to make them more filling. Add extra vegetables to starters or main dishes, such as stir fries, pasta dishes, and salads. Salads are a great low energy density food if not smothered with high fat dressings so aim for low fat salad dressings, such as those based on lemon juice or vinegar and always ask for dressing on the side if eating out.

▸ Moderate the portion size when choosing any foods from the 'medium energy density' category (1.5 to 4 calories/gram). These foods include many sandwiches, pizza, lasagne, steak, curries, and chips.

▸ Not surprisingly, foods with a high energy density (more than 4 calories/gram) tend to be high in fat and have a low water content, for example biscuits and confectionery, crisps, peanuts, crackers, cheese, butter, oil, and mayonnaise. If you are following a low energy density diet, you can still eat foods from this category, but in small portions and not too often. Avoid using too much oil or butter in cooking and aim to use only a little butter or mayonnaise in sandwiches. You could also use reduced fat mayonnaise as an alternative.

▸ Add extra fruit to desserts and use cream sparingly. You could use low fat yogurt or fromage frais as an alternative to cream.

▸ 'Sugary drinks' includes fruit juices so you should limit your daily amount to no more than 150ml, which is one of your five-a-day. You should at least limit your intake of sugar-sweetened drinks to no more than 450 calories/36oz per week, according to the American Heart Association.[29]

What about glycemic index and glycemic load?

You may have heard of these indexes, which measure how particular foods affect blood sugar levels. The glycemic index

(GI) compares equal weights of carbohydrate and provides a measure of carbohydrate *quality*, but not *quantity*. In 1997 the concept of glycemic load (GL) was introduced by researchers at Harvard University to assess the overall effect on blood sugar levels of a typical serving of food. The higher the GL, the greater the expected elevation in blood glucose and insulin levels. For example, a 120g punnet of raspberries, strawberries, or blueberries is 1GL, whereas a banana is 12GL. A long-term high GL diet is associated with an increased risk of Type 2 diabetes and heart disease.[30] These authors published an 'International Table of GI and GL values' in the *American Journal of Clinical Nutrition*, although we would suggest you have a look at books by Patrick Holford if you want to know more about these values. He has written extensively on the subject, including recipe books and handy booklets you can carry around with you. Following a low GL diet is a way of keeping your blood sugar steady so that you avoid the daily 'peaks and troughs' caused by a high intake of sugar and refined carbohydrates.

What is the evidence?

In an Italian study, women with breast cancer were interviewed over three years and average daily GI and GL were calculated from a food frequency questionnaire. High GI foods, such as white bread, increased the risk of breast cancer while the intake of pasta, a medium GI food, seemed to have no influence (Augustin *et al.* 2001).[31] A further study indicated that a higher dietary GL may be a risk factor for endometrial cancer incidence in nondiabetic women.[32]

When it comes to fruits and vegetables, is 'five a day' enough?

Most of us are aware that fruit, vegetables, and fibre are cancer-protective. Five is a minimum recommended amount set by the government. However, health experts believe the optimum amount should be two to three fruits and six to eight vegetables per day. Pigments that give fruits and vegetables their colour contain a variety of protective compounds (see Table 2.1), for your immune system and to protect against cancer and heart disease.

Antioxidants

As explained in Chapter 1, low-density lipoprotein (LDL) cholesterol is only 'bad' when it is oxidised. Oxidised means a chemical reaction has happened, involving oxygen, such as when oxygen causes iron to rust, or an apple to go brown when exposed to the air. Oxidised LDL can be prevented by making sure you have a good supply of antioxidants in your diet, such as beta-carotene, vitamins C and E, zinc (oysters, meat, nuts and seeds, and grains) and selenium (nuts and seeds, seafood, meat, and grains). Fresh fruit and vegetables contain many vitamins and antioxidants, which may also help prevent dementia and heart disease. Table 2.1 shows the different protective compounds in different coloured fruits and vegetables and the benefits of including them in your diet.

TABLE 2.1 PROTECTIVE COMPOUNDS IN FRUIT AND VEGETABLES

Colour	Protective compound	Food sources	What they do
Red	Lycopene	Tomatoes, watermelon, guava	Antioxidant; cuts cancer risk
Orange	Beta-carotene	Carrots, yams, sweet potatoes, mangos, pumpkins	Antioxidant; supports immune system
Yellow-orange	Vitamin C Flavonoids	Oranges, lemons, grapefruits, papaya, peaches	Detoxifies harmful substances, inhibits tumour cell growth
Green	Folate Indoles	Spinach, broccoli, kale, Brussels sprouts	Eliminates excess oestrogens and carcinogens; builds healthy cells and DNA
Green-white	Indoles Lutein	Cabbage, cauliflower	Eliminates excess oestrogens and carcinogens
White-green	Allyl sulfides	Garlic, onions, asparagus, chives	Destroys cancer cells, supports immune system
Red-purple	Resveratrol	Grapes, berries, plums	Can help to balance oestrogen production and elimination
Blue	Anthocyanins	Blueberries, purple grapes, plums	Antioxidant

What is a healthy diet?

Adopting a healthy and balanced diet for life will help you to maintain a healthy body weight, and reduce your likelihood of developing high blood pressure or heart disease, both of which can put you at greater risk of developing dementia. It's fine to treat yourself occasionally but aim to eat healthily and moderate your fat intake most of the time.

A Mediterranean style diet may help reduce the risk of dementia, cancer, heart disease, and many other conditions and is relatively easy to follow. This diet typically has a high proportion of fish, fruit, vegetables, and unsaturated fat, and a low proportion of dairy products, meat, and saturated fat. Sources of unsaturated fat include oily fish, nuts, seeds, and olive oil.

What does 'limit alcoholic drinks' actually mean?

Although red wine has been shown to cut the risk of heart disease, for cancer prevention the optimum level is zero. The WCRF panel agreed that the levels set for minimum heart risk should be accepted, which are no more than two units a day for men and one for women.

UK government advice in 1995 was that regular consumption of two to three units a day for women (three to four for men), would not pose significant health risks. However, new guidelines issued at the beginning of 2016 are that men and women who drink regularly should consume no more than 14 units a week. The latest guidance makes it clear that people should be teetotal on some days, that heavy drinking sessions should be avoided, and also that no level of drinking is completely safe. The UK's chief medical officers say new research shows any amount of alcohol can increase the risk of cancer. Many people get confused as to how much a unit is, as this can vary depending on the type and strength of the alcohol. The strength is usually listed as a percentage ABV, which stands for Alcohol by Volume. It is important to know this figure when calculating the number of units you consume per week.

Wine: A glass of wine can contain anything from around one-and-a-half to three units, depending on the size of the glass and the strength of the wine.

▶ a medium glass (175ml) of 12% ABV: 2 units

▶ a large glass (250ml) of 12% ABV: 3 units

▶ a 750ml bottle of 12%: 9 units

▶ a 750ml bottle of 16%: 12 units

▶ a 750ml bottle of port 20%: 15 units.

Beer and cider:

▶ a pint of 4%-strength beer: 2.3 units

▶ a pint of 5%-strength beer: 2.8 units

▶ a pint of strong cider (8%): 4.5 units.

Spirits:

▶ a small glass (25ml)/40% ABV: 1 unit

▶ a small glass (50ml) of sherry, fortified wine or cream liqueur: 1 unit.

Drinking above these recommended levels significantly increases the risk of Alzheimer's, vascular dementia, and various cancers. A review of evidence indicates that moderate to heavy consumption of alcohol increases the risk of developing cancer of the oral cavity and pharynx, oesophagus, stomach, larynx, colorectum, pancreas, breast, and prostate. However, this same review did not find any association between alcohol consumption and an increased risk of cancers of the lung, bladder, endometrium, and ovary.[33] Even light drinking increases the risk of cancer of oral cavity and pharynx, oesophagus, and breast.[34] In a large study of health professionals in the US, it was found that the risk of alcohol related cancers (mainly breast cancer) increases even within the range of up to one alcoholic drink a day.[35]

Food intolerances

A food allergy normally causes symptoms within a few minutes of eating the offending food or being in contact with the relevant substance and will most likely have been present since birth. Because true food allergies cause an immune reaction, most adults will already be aware if they have an allergy to a particular food. Common food allergens include fish (including shellfish), eggs, and peanuts.

With a food intolerance (non-allergic hypersensitivity), the onset of symptoms is usually slower and may be delayed by many hours after eating the offending food. Symptoms may also last for many hours, even into the next day.

In some people, certain foods and drinks can trigger a migraine. One well accepted migraine trigger is tyramine, a substance found naturally in some foods, especially aged and fermented foods, such as:

▶ aged chicken liver

▶ aged cheese

▶ cured meats

▶ red wine

▶ sauerkraut

▶ smoked fish

▶ some types of beer

▶ soy sauce.

Food allergies can be determined by blood or skin tests. However, food intolerances are much more difficult to test for and, although there are some very sophisticated tests available, they are expensive. Therefore, the best way to determine if a particular food is an issue for you is to keep a diary (see Chapter 6), including the foods you've eaten during the past day or two (remember that symptoms may not occur for 24 hours after you eat certain trigger foods). The most accurate way of identifying whether food intolerance is contributing to migraines, or another health condition, is to exclude the suspected foods, in a controlled way, and then re-introduce them individually and monitor any effects (called an Elimination and Challenge Diet). This should ideally take place after a consultation with a specialist as elimination diets must be followed strictly, and for the correct period of time, to be effective. There are many books on the subject, or you can consult a nutrition expert if you need assistance in this area. Please note that it is not advisable to exclude large groups of foods without seeking advice from a specialist.

What about our environment?

Every day we are exposed to thousands of different chemicals and pollutants in the environment and some can have an effect on our hormones and overall health.

Endocrine disrupting chemicals (EDCs)

As explained in the last chapter, EDCs are chemicals, or combinations of chemicals, that interfere with any aspect of human hormonal action. They can be found in everything from pharmaceuticals to many common household items. Examples include:

▶ perfluorochemicals (PFCs), used as an ingredient to make products that resist heat, oil, stains, grease, and water. Common uses include non-stick cookware, stain-resistant carpets and fabrics (e.g. oil and water repellents for leather, paper, and textiles), coatings on some food packaging, and fire-fighting foams

▶ Bisphenol A (BPA), used in many everyday items, such as plastic bottles (now banned in baby bottles) and containers, linings for canned foods (to prevent corrosion), eye glass lenses, household appliances, cars, and planes; medical equipment, detergents, toys, even cash receipts have been reported to contain high levels (if on thermal receipt paper). BPA has been linked to Type 2 diabetes, insulin resistance, breast cancer, and uterine cancer in women

▶ pesticides

▶ surfactants – glue, plastic, rubber, paint, and wood products.

The list is endless so we won't include them all. Exposure to EDCs has been linked to increased incidence of certain cancers, cardiovascular disease, reduced sperm quality, earlier age of puberty, declines in fertility rates, increased rates of pregnancy complications, and developmental problems in humans. There is a great deal of research and ongoing debate in this area. The late Theo Colborn, an environmental health analyst, best known for her studies on the health effects of

EDCs, received many awards for her work in this area. In 2003, she founded The Endocrine Disruption Exchange (TEDX), an organisation devoted to understanding how EDCs interfere with development and health. This was after she wrote one of the most well-known books on the subject.[36] Please see the TEDX website if you are interested in finding out more.

How do I reduce my exposure to EDCs?

Since these chemicals are prevalent in everyday living, there is no way to avoid exposure completely. However, there are a number of ways to reduce exposure. For example, although it is almost impossible to avoid plastics completely, you can at least limit your use of them and be aware of which are the safest plastics:

▸ You can tell if your bottle contains BPA by looking at the recycling symbol on the bottom of it and the number within that triangle (usually above the letters PET or PETE, HDPE, LDPE, or PVC) ranging from 1 to 7. These symbols indicate how toxic the chemicals used in the plastic are, how likely the plastic is to leach, how bio-degradable the plastic is, and ultimately the safety of the plastic.

▸ Plastic bottles with the numbers 1, 2, 4, and 5 are generally regarded as safe. Number 1 (PET or PETE) is generally regarded as a safe plastic and the plastic mostly used for bottled water. However, it is not advisable to reuse any plastic bottle as they can get small, even unnoticeable, cracks in them which can cause them to leach out toxins.

▶ Avoid numbers 3, 6, and 7. Number 7 has been shown to be the greatest concern, with reports that this type of plastic can leach a toxin that has been linked to breast and ovarian cancer.

▶ Even the so-called 'good' plastics can leach chemicals when heated, so never put warm or hot liquid into any water bottle or plastic container, and don't microwave in plastic containers (transfer to a microwave safe bowl).

Other ways to reduce exposure to harmful chemicals:

▶ Buy organic wherever possible, not just food but personal care products and paints as well.

▶ Wash hands frequently, especially before you eat.

▶ Buy food and drink, wherever possible, in glass or ceramic containers instead of plastic or cans.

▶ Always choose fragrance-free products.

▶ Avoid, or at least limit, canned food, especially acidic foods like tomatoes. Buy either in BPA-free cans or glass containers where possible.

▶ Filters containing activated carbon, such as brita filters, can filter out many chemicals, including PFCs. If you install a water filter treatment unit at home, make sure you use a reliable installer to insure proper installation, operation, and maintenance of the system.

▶ Fish from all sources can contain contaminants, so it is good to be careful about the kinds of fish you eat and how often.

What are governments doing to reduce our exposure?

There are constant debates about how regulators should assess the risks of these potentially dangerous chemicals.

The European Food Safety Authority (EA) published a report at the beginning of 2015, concluding that there is no health concern for BPA at the estimated levels of dietary and non-dietary sources combined. However, the EA Panel noted that there is a considerable uncertainty in the exposure estimate for non-dietary sources.[37] Much more research needs to be done to determine how EDCs affect endocrine function and how exposure may affect future disease incidence.

Chapter 2 summary

In this chapter, we have covered basic principles that relate to our health, whatever our age. To summarise:

▶ Be physically active, as lean as possible within the normal range of body weight, and avoid weight gain throughout adulthood.

▶ Include omega-3s in your diet every day (two to three servings of fish each week, preferably oily; and nuts, seeds, seaweed, and soy).

▶ Limit sugar as much as possible and keep your blood sugar level as stable as possible throughout the day, by following a low energy dense, or low-GL diet.

▶ Aim for two to ten portions of fruits and vegetables daily (two to three fruits and six to seven vegetables). They contain a variety of protective compounds, such as antioxidants, for your immune system and to protect against cancer and heart disease.

▶ A Mediterranean style diet is a good example of a healthy diet (a high proportion of fish, fruit, vegetables, and unsaturated fat (oily fish, nuts, seeds, olive oil) and a low proportion of dairy products, meat, and saturated fat.

▶ Although red wine has been shown to cut the risk of heart disease, for cancer prevention the optimum level is zero. Drinking above recommended levels (no more than two units a day for men and one for women) significantly increases the risk of Alzheimer's, vascular dementia, and various cancers.

▶ Follow the guidelines on page 65 on how to reduce your exposure to endocrine disrupting chemicals (EDCs).

In the next chapter we will explore nutrients that have been specifically researched in relation to menopause, including those that can be taken in supplement form. We will also detail the herbs on the market that claim to reduce or alleviate the symptoms of the menopause and help you reduce your risk of associated health conditions, as outlined in Chapter 1.

Chapter 3

NUTRITION AND DIETARY SUPPLEMENTS FOR THE MENOPAUSE

The internet and high street are awash with health food stores that offer a vast array of products to deal with our ills and advice on what we should eat at various points in our lives. Some of the preparations found in health food retailers and online have a sound basis in scientific research with regard to their mechanism of action (how they work) and conditions they benefit. However, many do not and although this might not necessarily mean that the products don't have some health-giving properties, they have yet to be tested with the rigour demanded by researchers and large-scale health bodies such as the NHS and National Institute of Health (NIH) in the United States. Hence, you or someone you know (and online support groups) may have found symptomatic relief with a particular supplement or herb but, in this chapter as throughout this book, we will focus on the preparations that have been studied in the greatest of detail. This is not to imply that these are the only products on the market, rather the supplements discussed here are the ones grounded in research evidence. In this chapter, we will cover the benefits and safety of phytoestrogens, herbal remedies, and other nutrients that are specifically related to menopause or associated health conditions.

Phytoestrogens

Phytoestrogens are natural compounds, found in plant foods. The most important dietary groups of phytoestrogens are called isoflavones and lignans. The major isoflavones are genistein and daidzein, found in beans and pulses, particularly soya beans and soy products; chick peas; and red clover. Lignans are found in flaxseeds (the richest source), and also in many cereals, fruits, vegetables, and legumes.

What are phytoestrogens?

Phytoestrogens have a similar chemical structure to oestradiol and are therefore able to mimic the action of the body's own oestrogen, although they can have different effects in different parts of the body. This is because there are two different types of oestrogen receptors (ERs): ER beta, found predominantly in bone and blood vessels; and ER alpha, found predominantly in breast and womb tissue.[38] A receptor is the part of the cell where a chemical binds to the cell and 'locks on', a bit like a 'lock and key' mechanism. As with the different forms of oestrogen (oestradiol, oestrone, oestriol), phytoestrogens also bind differently to the different receptors, which means that oestrogen levels can be increased where needed most (as in bones and to reduce menopausal symptoms for example), and decreased if levels are high and could prove dangerous, as in breast or womb tissue. There is evidence that phytoestrogens are particularly beneficial for hormone-dependent diseases such as breast and prostate cancers and osteoporosis.[39]

They have been extensively researched, partly because vasomotor symptoms are much less frequently experienced by Asian women than by women in the West and some believe the Asian diet being rich in phytoestrogens may be a contributing factor to this lack of symptom occurrence.[40] Evidence suggests that about 10 per cent of the Asian population consumes as much as 25g of soy protein or 100mg of isoflavones per day.[41] In contrast, it is estimated that 1–3mg of isoflavones are consumed per day by the average person in the UK.

Soya

Soya has been widely promoted as a superfood that can fight breast cancer, strengthen bones, and ease the menopause. It is an excellent source of protein and the British Nutrition Foundation recommends adding traditional soya-bean products such as tofu, tamari, miso, and tempeh to a healthy and varied diet. The word 'traditional' is key, as sources such as tofu, miso, tempeh, and natto are fermented and the type consumed in Asian populations; whereas the type of soya generally consumed in the West is often highly processed. Foods containing soya include breakfast cereals, cereal bars, dairy and bakery products, soups, and sauces – the list goes on. It is used to add flavour, bulk, and texture to foods (it is estimated to be found in 60 per cent of processed foods) and can appear on food labels as 'hydrolysed/textured vegetable protein', 'soy protein isolate', 'plant sterols', or the emulsifier 'lecithin'.

Like most foods that are good for us, you can have too much of a good thing. Soya is healthy in small quantities, but could be unhealthy if eaten in excess. One small portion, about 30–40g a day, is ideal.

Benefits
VASOMOTOR SYMPTOMS

There have been many attempts to assess the effects of phytoestrogens by grouping together results from all studies but this has proved difficult as the studies are very different when it comes to participant numbers, ages, doses, and type of preparations used, and outcomes being measured.[42] Two reviews, one in 2009[43] and one in 2013,[44] were unable to reach a conclusion on whether phytoestrogens truly help with vasomotor symptoms. However, the very latest review[45] points out that three of the studies included in the 2013 review reported a reduction in the frequency of hot flushes from the use of soy extracts of between 21 and 43 per cent. We would guess that if you had been one of those women experiencing a 21–43 per cent reduction in hot flushes, you would be pretty relieved, especially if your symptoms were mild to moderate.

When it comes to assessing the effects on vasomotor symptoms in studies, some have measured the frequency of hot flushes, whereas others measured the severity of not just hot flushes, but other menopausal symptoms as well, to give a more rounded assessment of the experience of menopausal symptoms. One measure of 11 different symptoms is called the Kupperman index.

The Kupperman index

The Kupperman index (KI) is a numerical index used in some studies to score not just hot flushes, but also 10 other symptoms, such as paraesthesia, insomnia, nervousness, melancholia, vertigo, weakness, arthralgia, or myalgia, headache, palpitations, and formication (an abnormal skin sensation like insects crawling over, or within, the skin). Each symptom is rated from zero (no symptoms) to three (most severe) and the total sum calculated.

In the most recent review, of 15 high-quality studies, three of the seven studies that used this index reported a significant reduction in the phytoestrogen group, while the other four reported no difference between the groups. When they pooled the seven studies together, no significant treatment effect of phytoestrogen compared to placebo was found. This shows the importance of looking at individual studies. When it came to looking at hot flush frequency in a total of ten studies, four reported a significant reduction of hot flush frequency in the phytoestrogen group, while the other six reported no significant difference between the groups. However, pooling the data from these ten studies indicated that the phytoestrogen group had a significant reduction in hot flush frequency compared with the placebo group.[46]

As stated above, it is sometimes difficult to reach a conclusion on whether phytoestrogens truly help with vasomotor symptoms. Having said that, phytoestrogens have very few, if any, side effects and some women may benefit from a reduction in hot flushes, and possibly other menopausal symptoms.

The placebo effect

The American anaesthesiologist Henry K. Beecher was the first researcher to scientifically quantify this now very well-known phenomenon of symptom reduction arising from the belief that a treatment will reduce symptoms, and not the result of an active substance. In his 1955 article 'The Powerful Placebo', Beecher reported that 35 per cent of over a thousand patients suffering from various conditions (from post-operative wound pain to the common cold) had recovered from dummy pills and solutions alone.[47] In modern-day medical research, studies that aim to prove the effectiveness of a particular treatment will usually include a 'placebo group', where a comparable group of people will be given either a placebo pill (which will be made to look, smell, and even taste like the active medication) in order to make sure that any improvements seen following treatment are due to the treatment itself, and not the placebo effect. Even studies that don't investigate substances will include a placebo group; for instance research into psychological therapies will include a comparison therapy or technique that's similar in terms of the time a patient spends with a therapist and the therapy's activities to make sure that it's not simply the process of going through an intervention (known as an 'intervention effect'), but rather the key characteristics of the therapy that produces positive changes. Hence a person's belief that a treatment can make them better can itself be the active ingredient and cause symptom change, which is why throughout this book there are many instances of symptom reduction in the placebo groups of cited research studies.

BREAST AND ENDOMETRIAL HEALTH

Studies suggest that soya food intake in the amount consumed in Asian populations may have protective effects against breast and endometrial cancer, and teenagers and young adults who consume relatively high levels of phytoestrogens are less likely to develop aggressive forms of breast cancer when they reach middle age. Asian women consuming 20mg or more of dietary isoflavones daily had a 29 per cent reduction in breast cancer risk, compared with those consuming less than 5mg daily.[48] Chinese population studies have also reported that regular intake of soya foods is associated with a reduced risk of endometrial cancer, particularly among women with a higher BMI or waist:hip ratio.[49] It should be noted, however, that the majority of Asian women included in these studies have most likely had regular amounts of soy in their diet throughout childhood and adolescence and it is a matter of debate as to whether the same benefits apply if intake is only increased in adulthood in Western women.

Safety

It is thought unlikely that consuming isoflavones at dietary levels of less than 100mg daily could have breast cancer-promoting effects in healthy women, or breast cancer survivors not undergoing treatment. However, breast cancer patients receiving treatment may need to limit dietary soya intake and avoid isoflavone supplements, based on findings from one animal study showing that genistein may interfere with tamoxifen treatment if taken at the same time.[50]

The long-term safety of phytoestrogens with regard to the endometrium (womb lining) was called into question after a five-year study with soy phytoestrogens (150mg per day) was associated with an increased occurrence of endometrial hyperplasia (thickening of womb lining that may develop into cancer).[51] However, a more recent trial showed no difference in endometrial thickness, or cancer, in women receiving an isoflavone supplement (154mg per day) for three years, compared to women taking dummy pills.[52] It is puzzling why such high doses were used in these studies, considering that only 10 per cent of Asian women are estimated to consume up to 100mg per day of dietary isoflavones.[53] We would not recommend a daily intake of higher than 100mg, to included dietary sources and supplements.

HEART HEALTH

Soya has been shown to reduce 'bad' low-density lipoprotein (LDL) cholesterol and increase 'good' high-density lipoprotein (HDL) cholesterol in many studies. The US Food and Drug Administration recommends at least 25g of soy protein each day, as this is the amount that has been shown to lower cholesterol.

Possible negative effects of phytoestrogens on thyroid function

It is possible that a high intake of soya might interfere with thyroid function and disrupt hormones, leading to weight gain, fatigue, and mood problems. This is because soya can block the uptake of iodine, which is needed for a healthy thyroid. Soya contains goitrogens, which are naturally-occurring substances found in various other foods, such as Brussels sprouts, cauliflower, cabbage, kale, almonds, peanuts, walnuts, swede, and turnips. They can prevent the thyroid from using available iodine and have the ability to cause a goiter, which is an enlargement of the thyroid gland. This can also be made worse if you consume a lot of salt because that can cause the thyroid to swell. Fortunately, you don't have to give up these foods completely as the enzymes involved in the formation of goitrogenic materials in plants can be at least partially destroyed by heat, so you can still enjoy these foods when steamed or cooked. This is very important to consider if you consume a lot of raw food and/or juice raw vegetables, such as cabbage and spinach, as overconsumption of raw goitrogens may be able to slow down the thyroid, and/or promote development of a goiter. You should not eat these foods in large amounts, especially if you have a thyroid condition and are taking medication for it. If you have been diagnosed with a thyroid problem, you will have been told to restrict your intake of all these foods. However, a three-year

. trial set up specifically to assess the effects of genestein .
: (54 mg/day) on thyroid function showed that genistein :
: did not increase the risk of hypothyroidism.[54] So, if you :
: don't have a thyroid problem, you can still enjoy these :
: foods (preferably cooked) and don't consume these foods :
: raw in large quantities. :

Red clover

Red clover (*trifolium pratense*) is the richest source of natural isoflavones, containing genistein, daidzein (as with soya), but also formononetin and biochanin. Promensil is an extract of red clover used in some studies (see below). Each tablet contains 40mg of isoflavones, and the most common dosages used in trials are 40–80mg daily. We should warn you that not all red clover products are the same. A UK survey of 35 supplements found that only 14 contained the required 40mg minimum effective level of isoflavones, with six delivering less than 10mg.[55] You should check with your doctor if you are on any kind of medication as some types of red clover may contain coumarins, which could interfere with blood clotting and have the potential for interacting with some medications. However, some commercially available supplements, including Promensil and Rimostil, have been analysed to ensure that there are no coumarins present.[56]

Benefits
HOT FLUSHES

A dose of 80mg of Promensil, taken for 12 weeks, resulted in a 44 per cent reduction in both the frequency and severity of hot flushes, although the lower dose of 40mg was not effective.[57] Other studies have also shown a reduction in the number of hot flushes after 12–16 weeks of supplementing with red clover isoflavones.[58]

BONE HEALTH

Promensil (40mg per day) reduced the loss of bone mineral density (BMD) in the lumbar spine after one year and there was also a beneficial effect on bone quality.[59] Another study reported higher BMD for femoral neck and lumbar spine in genistein-treated women.[60]

HEART HEALTH

Isoflavones from red clover have been shown to be protective for the heart by reducing total cholesterol and 'bad' (LDL) cholesterol levels and increasing 'good' (HDL) cholesterol in a 12-month trial.[61] Furthermore, a red clover supplement, at doses of both 40mg and 80mg, was found to have a beneficial effect on arterial compliance, which is a measurement of the elasticity of large arteries.[62]

DEPRESSION/ANXIETY

Red clover (80mg daily for 90 days) was found to be effective in reducing depressive and anxiety symptoms among postmenopausal women.[63]

Safety
BREAST AND ENDOMETRIAL HEALTH

To date, there is no evidence to suggest that red clover may affect the breast or the endometrium in a negative way, although long-term studies are lacking and larger trials are needed to evaluate this. However, trials so far, lasting up to 3 years, do not show any negative effects on either the breast[64] or the endometrium.[65]

How do phytoestrogens compare with HRT?

Only a few studies have compared the effect of phytoestrogens or soy products with HRT. The British Menopause Society reported in 2013 that vasomotor symptoms reduce up to a maximum of 60 per cent when taking phytoestrogens, compared to 90–100 per cent with traditional HRT.[66]

However, a study comparing low-dose hormone therapy to a daily isoflavone supplement showed a similar reduction in hot flushes in both groups. Patients who received the isoflavone supplement experienced a 49.8 per cent reduction, compared to those on low-dose HRT, where the reduction was 45.6 per cent.[67]

Vitamins and minerals

Vitamin D and calcium

These two nutrients are difficult to separate, especially when it comes to bone health. The role of calcium for healthy bones and teeth is well known, although it has many other uses including regulating heartbeat, and ensuring that blood clots normally. Low levels of vitamin D have been associated with an increased risk of death from heart disease, cognitive impairment in older adults, and cancer, and could also play a role in the prevention and treatment of a number of different conditions, including diabetes and high blood pressure. There is no doubt that calcium does slow postmenopausal bone loss and vitamin D is needed for the correct absorption of calcium. However, the two nutrients must be in balance and an excess of vitamin D can have a negative effect on calcium balance. Stress levels can also affect our bones, since calcium is continually being moved out of and into the blood stream, in response to hormones which regulate our body's needs.

When considering calcium and vitamin D for preventing fractures, it would appear that they need to be combined to have an effect as vitamin D taken alone has not been shown to be effective in studies.[68] However, calcium and vitamin D supplementation has recently been associated with an increased risk of heart attacks, strokes, kidney stones, gastrointestinal symptoms, and admissions to hospital with acute gastrointestinal problems.[69, 70] Therefore current recommendations are to obtain calcium from the diet in preference to supplements,[71] although some people may not consume calcium in high enough levels from diet alone. Have a look at the foods below and be sure to include them in good quantities in your diet.

Good food sources

Calcium: dairy products, fish (especially sardines and pilchards if you eat the bones), green leafy vegetables, soya and kidney beans, tofu, nuts and seeds, brown rice, wholemeal bread, and anything made with fortified flour.

Vitamin D: Fish (particularly oily fish) and fish oils, egg yolks, cheese, fortified milk, liver, and some meat. Because most food sources are animal-based, you may become deficient if you follow a vegetarian or vegan diet and may have to supplement if tests show your level is low.

Some experts recommend that supplements should only be taken by those with risk factors and if test results reveal low levels.[72] Risk factors include not gaining enough of these nutrients from diet alone or, in the case of vitamin D, lack of sunlight; having a darker skin (because more time is required in the sun to gain the same benefits as a person with fairer skin); and frailty, which is often associated with less time in the sun and/or poor diet. Vitamin D has also been found to be low in all Northern Hemisphere countries in the winter months. If you are in any doubt, you should see your doctor and get your levels tested. In young, healthy individuals, a blood level of 50nmol/l or above is considered 'sufficient', although some experts believe that the optimum level is at least 75nmol/l in relation to most health outcomes, including bone mineral density (BMD) and lower risk of fractures; and for cancer prevention, desirable levels are between 90–120nmol/l.[73]

Take home message for vitamin D and calcium

▶ Calcium has many important uses in the body and vitamin D deficiency has been associated with many health conditions.

▶ It is important to test vitamin D levels and to supplement if deficient, under the guidance of a health professional.

▶ When it comes to preventing fractures, vitamin D used alone does not appear to be effective. However, when combined with calcium, it has been effective in some studies but not all.

▶ High calcium intakes have been associated with an increased risk of heart attacks, kidney stones, and gastrointestinal problems so it is important to consider your dietary intake and consult a health professional before taking supplements.

▶ If you are at risk of osteoporosis and are considering supplementing calcium and vitamin D, it is best to do so as part of a bone-building/protection formula or under the guidance of your doctor or nutritional therapist.

Other vitamins and minerals for bone health

One very important factor to consider when supplementing any vitamin or mineral is that they work synergistically – that is, they require other vitamins and minerals for their correct function (called co-factors). For example, calcium requires vitamin D for proper absorption and other vitamins, such as vitamin K, as well as a number of minerals to ensure that it is incorporated into bone rather than other body tissues (such as the heart). In addition to calcium and vitamin D, the majority of bone-building, or bone protection, formulas also contain vitamin K, magnesium, zinc, boron, and manganese, amongst others. If you have any of the risk factors for osteoporosis, as detailed in Chapter 1, please consult a nutrition expert who will be able to advise you further.

Evening primrose oil

Evening primrose oil is derived from the seeds of the evening primrose plant (*Oenothera biennis*) and comprises a good source of polyunsaturated fatty acid (PUFA) particularly gamma-linolenic acid (GLA) and linoleic acid. PUFAs are important in health and wellbeing throughout life and in particular protect against heart disease, inflammatory disease, and osteoporosis.[74] Animals, including humans, cannot produce GLA so we must access this PUFA from our food (linseeds are exceptionally high in GLA) or via supplementation. When taken within recommended dosages, evening primrose oil is safe and generally well tolerated.

Evening primrose oil has not been researched as extensively as black cohosh for alleviating the symptoms of the menopause, but there is some evidence to support its use. One study with 56 women observed more improvements in hot flush severity in women taking 500mg twice a day of the supplement for six weeks than a placebo capsule.[75]

However, both the evening primrose group and the placebo group saw improvements in hot flush frequency, severity, and duration and also the amount that this symptom interfered with daily life (the *placebo effect* is explained earlier in this chapter). Furthermore, the women taking evening primrose oil reported less intrusion from hot flushes in social activities, interpersonal relations and sexual functioning than those in the placebo group.

However, an earlier study did not find these beneficial effects, although there was a reduction in the total number of night time hot flushes in women who were given evening primrose supplements compared to a placebo.[76] Nevertheless, many thousands of women do use this supplement which ranks third behind herbal medicine and soya/phytoestrogens in terms of popularity when compared to other alternative and complementary healthcare options for menopausal symptoms.[77]

Take home message for evening primrose oil

▶ This is a commonly used supplement even though the evidence for its effectiveness for specific menopausal symptoms is lacking.

▶ Evening primrose oil is safe and may help with other health complaints relevant to menopausal women such as cardiovascular disease and osteoporosis.

Herbs

Black cohosh

This North American herb (*Cimicifuga racemosa*) of which the root and rhizome are used in preparations, has attracted a good deal of attention in the research community when considering it for dealing with the symptoms of the menopause. However, like many non-pharmacological treatments, the quality of the research studies can at best said to be mixed and some controversy reigns on black cohosh's efficacy. In a 2008 review of the evidence, six studies were identified which included over a thousand women.[78] The criteria for inclusion in this review were strict and studies that lacked a comparison group, contained data from women with medically-induced menopause, used preparations that mixed black cohosh with other substances, or did not focus primarily on menopausal symptoms were excluded. The authors of the review concluded that the weight of evidence was not strong enough to support the use of this herb for controlling the symptoms of the menopause. But there was a caveat to this conclusion in that there seemed to be a benefit of taking this herb for women who experience symptoms during the perimenopause.

A subsequent review by a different group of researchers published in 2012 found 16 studies (totalling 2027 individual women) that were of sufficient quality and met the same stringent criteria as the 2008 investigation into black cohosh and menopausal symptoms.[79] This study also did not find convincing evidence for the herb's effectiveness and in fact reported that HRT was better at reducing hot flushes and overall symptoms. Yet this analysis has been questioned and a further look at the body of research led a team of clinicians to dispute these claims of black cohosh's ineffectiveness stating that using this herb is more beneficial than taking a non-active substance (i.e. placebo).[80] Nevertheless, the way in which black cohosh works has not be established although initial concerns over its safety with regard to liver toxicity appear to have been refuted.[81,82,83] Possible interactions with medications may be an issue for some women so please do speak with your doctor before trying this herbal remedy.

Take home message for black cohosh

▶ If you are taking any other medicines, only use this remedy with medical guidance as there is no consensus on its safety although liver toxicity now seems unlikely.

▶ Black cohosh may benefit women during the perimenopause but there is not enough evidence at present to state this for certain, nor do we know exactly how it works.

St John's wort

St John's wort (*Hypericum perforatum*) is a herb that has been shown to be effective for mild to moderate depression in both peri- and premenopausal women. It works in a similar way to SSRIs (see next chapter), although the two should not be taken together.

St John's wort has also been found to be an effective treatment for vasomotor symptoms for perimenopausal and postmenopausal women. One study showed that the frequency, duration, and severity of hot flushes was reduced after eight weeks of treatment.[84] This is consistent with an earlier study, which reported that the incidence and severity of typical psychological, psychosomatic, and vasomotor symptoms were substantially improved in menopausal symptoms, including sexual wellbeing. Menopausal complaints diminished or disappeared completely in the majority of women (76.4 per cent by patient evaluation and 79.2 per cent by physician evaluation).[85] It has also been found to improve sleep problems and quality of life after three months of treatment.[86]

Another study found that a combination of black cohosh and St John's wort is superior to placebo in alleviating menopausal complaints, including the related psychological component. It interacts with other medications, so please consult your doctor if this is something you wish to take.[87]

Take home message for St John's wort

▶ St John's wort has been shown to be effective for mild to moderate depression.

▶ It has also been found to reduce the frequency, duration, and severity of hot flushes and improve psychological symptoms, sleep problems, and quality of life.

▶ Caution is required if you are on other medication.

Ginseng

The root of this perennial herb, native to Korea and China, is used extensively not only in Asia as it is a component of many American supplements. However, when examining the research on this herb it's important to note that the common name ginseng is used to describe a number of chemically different species of *Panax* (e.g. *Panex ginseng*, which is also known as Asian ginseng; and *Panex qinquefolium*, which is referred to as American ginseng). There are numerous active agents within ginseng (and they differ between the different species) such as ginsenosides, fatty acids, polysaccharides, peptides, polyacetylenic, and alcohols.[88] Ginseng is often marketed as a cognitive booster and for the prevention of dementia but the evidence for this is patchy.[89] In the USA particularly, ginseng is packaged as a supplement for cardiovascular health, but again the research is equivocal.[90]

In terms of evaluating the findings of ginseng on menopausal symptoms, one review identified four studies with adequate methods and reporting, i.e. having a comparison group, using standard measures, etc.[91] Across these four studies benefits were found in women taking ginseng in terms of sexual arousal, general menopausal symptoms, depression, and overall health compared to women in the placebo group. However, one study did not support the beneficial claims of ginseng for menopausal symptoms and overall, the number of studies and women taking part in these research trails was simply too small to draw firm conclusions. Ginseng does appear to be safe, with few adverse side effects, although vaginal bleeding did occur for some women taking the supplement.[92]

Take home message for ginseng

▶ There is not enough evidence for the use of ginseng in managing menopausal symptoms, though it's unlikely to cause harm.

▶ The mechanisms by which ginseng improves health are complex and still to be completely unravelled. Some studies have seen cognitive and cardiovascular benefits but others have not; in time we will know more about the way in which ginseng works and which species should be used for particular health issues.

Chinese herbal medicine (CHM)

Chinese herbal medicine (CHM) is a component of Traditional Chinese Medicine that might be used either by itself or in conjunction with other methods such as acupuncture and exercises that involve deep breathing and controlled movements such as tai chi and qi gong (see Chapter 5). CHM practitioners work on a case-by-case basis, i.e. personalised medicine, so there is not a set protocol for dealing with the symptoms of the menopause, *per se*. This makes researching CHM quite difficult as it's not possible to unpick which component herbs in themselves influence symptom change. Nevertheless, one small-scale study which compared CHM to HRT and a placebo control group found CHM to be more beneficial for menopausal symptoms than the placebo capsules and tinctures in reducing hot flushes.[93] However, HRT out-performed CHM as women taking orthodox HRT saw the greatest reduction in hot flushes after 12 weeks of treatment.

Dong quai

Although the practice of CHM is personalised, there has been some research conducted that looked at one particular Chinese herb thought to have oestrogenic effects known as dong quai (*Angelica sinensis*). Seventy-one postmenopausal women were given dong quai or a placebo substance for 24 weeks and asked about their symptoms before and after treatment.[94] Also, in order to test more objectively for oestrogenic effects, vaginal cells were investigated for signs of cellular ageing and an ultrasound was performed to look at endometrial thickness. The findings of these measures were disappointing however as there were no notable differences between either the more objective tests in this study or the subjective (questionnaire) ratings of menopausal symptoms. But when combined with other herbs the effectiveness of dong quai appears more promising.[95] However, it's important to note that in some preparations of dong quai photosensitivity can be a concern and interactions with blood thinning drugs such as warfarin and increased bleeding have been reported when using this herb. Please discuss taking this herb with your medical doctor if any of these issues are relevant to you.

Take home message for CHM

▸ Because CHM is individualised to each patient, in practice different women will receive different combinations and amounts of herbs in CHM capsules and tinctures. Therefore, figuring out the active substances is hard when trying to maintain the Traditional Chinese Medicine approach in research studies. At present it's not possible to say with any certainty that CHM offers substantial benefits to women experiencing menopausal symptoms.

▶ Dong quai, also known as angelica, does not appear to be effective in treating the symptoms of the menopause alone nor has it been shown to have observable estrogenic effects. More research needs to be conducted to see in what combinations with other Chinese herbs this botanical is useful for symptomatic women.

Chapter 3 summary

There are many of thousands of products and supplements on the market that claim to reduce or alleviate the symptoms of the menopause, although the evidence for these statements is often scarce or conflicting. We have therefore covered only those with the most evidence. Relatively little is known about the interactions certain preparations have with prescribed and over-the-counter medications and therefore it is advised that if you are already taking medication (either for the menopause or for an entirely separate health issue) you should not stop this medication or take supplements without consulting your doctor, or health specialist, first. In the next chapter we will explore some of the psychological and behavioural therapies which have been shown to help with the management of menopausal symptoms; you may want to consider using these in addition to the nutritional strategies presented here and the self-help techniques outlined in Chapter 6.

Chapter 4

PSYCHOLOGICAL AND BEHAVIOURAL INTERVENTIONS

In the previous two chapters we looked at nutrition and dietary changes that can be made to alleviate some of the symptoms associated with the menopause as well as supplements and herbal remedies that have been studied with regard to symptom reduction. We've mentioned a number of studies so far that have found placebo effects, that is people have shown improvements in symptoms even when they were not taking an active ingredient. This in itself demonstrates the interaction of cognitive processes and physiological mechanisms, a field known as psychoneuroimmunology, or PNI, which we will discuss in this chapter. Following on from this, we'll outline a number of psychological and behavioural therapies that have been investigated with regard to menopausal symptoms. As throughout this book, the focus will be on the methods that have been studied scientifically and to the greatest extent. Whilst the core of the techniques in this chapter is a psychological and behavioural change approach, the value of these treatments can go beyond psychological symptoms and so may act as an important adjunct component to other treatments that you may want to use for your symptoms. Finally, we present a guide to finding a qualified therapist in the techniques mentioned in this chapter.

Why are psychological therapies relevant to the menopause?

Both acute and chronic stress trigger a vast array of emotional, psychological, and physiological changes in our bodies. You may have heard of a concept called 'the fight or flight response' or the 'stress response'. This is when our bodies ready themselves to either go into battle with a real or perceived 'threat' by shifting energy and nutrients to our muscles and increasing our awareness. Think for a moment; if you hear a loud noise at night, your heart may start pounding, your hearing may seem more keen and your pupils may dilate. All of these physiological responses have been developed though evolution to give us the very best chances of survival, i.e. identify and stop an intruder or run if said intruder attacks. However, if our bodies' mechanisms cannot return to their natural resting state, health problems can occur. This influential theory was first conceptualised by Hans Seyle in the 1930s and now there are many tens of thousands of scientific studies devoted to study of stress and ill health.

How do psychological therapies help physical symptoms?

One area of research that blossomed in the field of health and stress is psychoneuroimmunology (PNI). Researchers and medics in this area have investigated how psychological and cognitive process can impact our state of health via the immune system. But they have also considered how immune activation and the process involved with our bodies' natural defences can in themselves alter our behaviour which, in turn, can also either trigger or reduce symptoms.[96,97] To give this idea some grounding, one study by eminent researchers Janice Kiecolt Glaser and Ronald Glaser and their teams selected a group of people under constant and profound stress – caregivers. People continually caring for others (often loved ones) experience intense emotional and psychological stress and sometimes physical stress too. So it is perhaps unsurprising that this group of people have been shown to be more susceptible to infectious disease and have slower healing times.[98]

Interestingly the relationship between stress and health is not one-way; experimental studies where participants were given substances that mimic an infection have shown that this can increase feelings of anxiety. Furthermore, stress does not just affect our immune systems. In menopausal women, stress may affect the thermoregulation system which is also controlled via the sympathetic nervous system (SNS) and thus therapeutic techniques that aim to reduce both chronic and acute stress may modify the experience of hot flushes and other common symptoms.[99] Therefore, there is a positive message here: we can influence our physical health via psychological means, such as relaxation, stress reduction techniques, and other 'talking' therapies. We will now look at these approaches in more detail.

Cognitive behavioural therapy (CBT)

Cognitive behavioural therapy (CBT) is a very well-known treatment that was developed by American psychiatrist Aaron Beck. Beck first conceptualised the idea of targeting unhelpful thoughts in response to his frustrations with existing techniques, particularly psychoanalytic therapy. Beck observed that many of his patients had quite negative views of themselves and the world around them, which appeared to play a part in their symptoms. Beck hypothesised that by guiding his patients to change these thoughts and beliefs (known as cognitions) and also the behaviours that maintained these, their situations would improve. CBT is now widely available and it has been evaluated robustly in many disorders defined as psychological or psychiatric[100] and also physical health problems.[101]

What is CBT?

CBT is a structured therapy, which usually consists of 6–12 sessions, although there is currently discussion on whether the treatment can be delivered in a single session. Before treatment starts an assessment will be carried out in order to pinpoint the specific difficulties an individual is having and the goals of the therapy (perhaps in the context of this book this would be symptom reduction). Then the therapist will guide the patient in an examination of her thought patterns and also explore the behaviours that may be associated with these cognitions. An example of an unhelpful thought pattern is 'My symptoms are completely ruining my life and I can't do anything properly any more' which may result in behaviours such as withdrawal from everyday social activities and even impact on relationships and work. CBT techniques work by reframing these cognitions into more beneficial and accurate thoughts which should then help patients to overcome difficulties and engage fully in life.

As CBT is essentially a process to change habits, it also generally requires 'homework' – that is, activities to do in between sessions to help develop the new and more constructive cognitions. These are not onerous however and can include something as simple as a diary to note down thoughts which can then be discussed in the next session. This therapy, like most psychological approaches, needs to be maintained even after the therapist sessions end, and so strategies to achieve this will also be discussed in the final CBT meetings.

CBT for menopausal symptoms

For some women hormone replacement therapies will not be appropriate, particularly those who have been diagnosed and treated for breast cancer because of concern over breast cancer reoccurring. Unfortunately, women who have had breast cancer tend to experience more severe menopausal symptoms, which can in turn affect sleep quality, mood, and general enjoyment of life.[102,103] Therefore, researchers have been looking at whether therapies like CBT can help to manage these symptoms.

One such study looked at patients who had more than ten episodes of night sweats or hot flushes a week following breast cancer treatment.[104] These women were invited to take part in six weekly sessions of group therapy, which included not only CBT techniques but also instruction on breathing techniques (see Chapters 4 and 6) and information about the symptoms of the menopause (outlined in Chapter 1). Therefore, the treatment that the women received was very much tailored to menopausal symptoms, rather than consisting of general CBT exercises. This group of women was compared to a group who only received their usual medical care. Nine weeks after the start of the study, the women who engaged in the group therapy had fewer problems with hot flushes and night sweats compared to women who only received standard medical care and these improvements lasted six-and-a-half months. There was a further knock-on effect as the women in the CBT group had fewer sleep problems than before they started treatment and also their mood and concentration levels improved. Finally, those in the therapeutic group said that they felt better able to deal with their symptoms in relation to work and social gatherings. Overall, from this study (and of course it is just one study but there are others that had similar promising findings) this non-hormonal and non-pharmacological treatment had notable and positive results for the women who participated in this form of talking therapy.

Self-help CBT

Although traditionally CBT is delivered on a one-to-one basis, over recent years there has been a surge of research looking at different ways to provide therapy and if these methods are as effective as individual therapy. This new, more flexible approach to the delivery of psychological therapy has occurred not only in menopause research but across the board and in a vast array of conditions. One study compared women who were given group-based CBT and what was termed as 'guided self-help CBT' (i.e. CBT that could be carried out at home independently rather than in a group) to a group of women who did not receive any form of treatment.[105] One hundred and forty symptomatic women took part in the study which assessed the women's estimation of troublesome night sweats and hot flushes six weeks after starting the therapies and also, like the group CBT study just mentioned, six-and-a-half months later to see if any beneficial effects remained. Improvements in these key menopausal symptoms were found in both the self-help and group CBT women at both time points. Furthermore, mood and overall quality of life improved in those women that had treatment. Hence, early evidence is illustrating that talking therapies don't necessarily need to be one-to-one or even face-to-face, which allows for a much greater flexibility and access to effective and supportive techniques for women who experience problematic symptoms during the menopause. There are many books on the market that explain in detail the techniques used in CBT which you may want to try in an effort to reduce symptoms, as this study has given some preliminary support for self-help CBT.

Take home message for CBT

▶ CBT is a safe treatment, particularly for women who cannot or do not want to use HRT.

▶ CBT appears to be effective at reducing the impact of menopausal symptoms not just in themselves but also with regard to sleep quality, daily life, and overall mood.

Hypnotherapy

Hypnotherapy, also known as clinical hypnosis, has a very long history and can be traced back to many ancient civilisations including the ancient Greek, Romans, and Egyptians and within Traditional Chinese Medicine. However, in terms of modern day history, Austrian physician Franz Anton Mesmer (1734–1815) is believed to be the founder of clinical hypnosis.[106] Although Mesmer's work involved the use of magnets to restore depleted levels of 'animal magnetism' he accepted that the magnets themselves were not curative; rather the interaction between the patient and hypnotist allowed for the former to transmit his magnetism to the patient. This of course is not modern-day practice but there were some clues in Mesmer's work that may explain how he helped his patients to recover from a range of ills, including the use of complex (and lengthy) hand gestures on the part of the hypnotist that perhaps helped his patients to enter into a state of deep relaxation.

What is hypnotherapy?

Like most talking or practitioner-guided therapies, hypnotherapy is the interaction between the instructions, or in this case 'suggestions', of the hypnotherapist which then enable the individual to focus their attention on inner sensations and experiences.[107] In this regard, a patient could not be 'made' or forced to enter a hypnotic state (sometimes called a 'trance') as she is always in total control over her thoughts and actions. Therefore hypnotherapy is better perceived as a type of guided, deep relaxation rather than a form of mind control.

In a hypnotherapy session, the practitioner will use a number of techniques such as progressive relaxation and the repetition of calming words or phrases to induce a hypnotic state. This state is similar to daydreaming; think about for instance when you've been totally fixed on a thought, so much so that you can't remember if you've carried out a certain action, perhaps washing your face in the shower or what you've gone into another room to retrieve. This is a type of hypnotic state as we are completely focused on our inner thoughts so our conscious is not attending to other information in our surroundings. The theory behind hypnotherapy is that while a person is in this hypnotic state, her mind is more open to change.

Clinical hypnosis has been shown to benefit numerous symptoms and health complaints including many different types of pain (e.g. acute and chronic pain[108] and headaches and migraine[109]) where the technique has been shown to be more effective than pain relief medication. In children, this type of therapy has also been shown to help in a range of conditions including headaches, abdominal pain, irritable bowel syndrome, insomnia, chronic eczema, and chemotherapy-related distress.[110] There are many theories and studies that suggest how hypnotherapeutic techniques produce analgesic effects including alterations in our central nervous system, specifically pathways that control blood pressure and heart rate, brain wave patterns, and the blood flow in the brain.[111]

Hypnotherapy for menopausal symptoms

In terms of hypnotherapy as a tool for the management of menopausal symptoms, a series of high quality studies, led by Gary Elkins, Professor of Psychology and Neuroscience and Director of the Mind-Body Medicine Research Laboratory at Baylor University in Texas, USA, have been conducted in recent years. In a small-scale preliminary study of 16 women who had experienced breast cancer, Dr Elkins and his colleagues found some very good results: after completing four weekly sessions of hypnosis, the women in this study reported a 59 per cent decrease in daily hot flushes and also a 70 per cent reduction in hot flushes on a weekly basis.[112] Improvements were also found in other areas such as work, social and leisure activities, sleep, mood, concentration, relationships, sexuality, and enjoyment of life. Based on these encouraging findings, Dr Elkins went onto carry out larger-scale research to further test this hypnotherapy technique which was specifically developed for this group of patients.

As Dr Elkins' first study did not have a comparison group, the next piece of research his team carried out compared women who participated in the hypnosis to women who had a similar medical history and symptom profile but did not receive any special treatment.[113] By the end of the five weeks of treatment, those in the hypnotherapy group had a 68 per cent reduction in hot flushes. The women in the control group had a slight decrease in symptoms but this was not seen as a clinical improvement. Of interest in this study, no one dropped out of the treatment group; in most drug studies people do drop out because of unpleasant side effects but this type of treatment, like CBT, does not produce unwanted symptoms. Also, a reduction of this magnitude is comparable to that of paroxetine and venlafaxine (see Chapter 9).

Further work by Dr Elkins and colleagues introduced a more comparable control group that received an intervention, rather than simply no additional treatment. This is important as sometimes the added time and attention from a therapist can produce positive findings, rather than improvements being due to the treatment itself. The comparison treatment in Elkins' next study consisted of 'attention control', which matched the clinical hypnosis sessions in every aspect except the hypnotic induction.[114] In other words, both groups received not just the same amount of time with a therapist but also had sessions within the same therapeutic environment and the level of therapist's encouragement was identical in both groups. Even better results were shown in this study as the women in the hypnotherapy group saw a 74 per cent reduction in hot flushes, whereas there was only a 17 per cent decrease in this symptom in the comparison group. Hence, it does appear that the hypnosis technique was indeed the 'active' ingredient in this series of studies after all. Sleep quality had also improved far more in the hypnotherapy group.

Take home message for hypnotherapy

▶ Like CBT, hypnotherapy is safe and doesn't cause worrisome side effects like some medications can (although it appears to be as effective as some drugs for treating menopausal symptoms).

▶ Hypnotherapy can also help to improve sleep, concentration, and ability to engage in wider social and personal activities.

Other psychological therapies for the treatment of menopausal symptoms

Over the past decade a therapeutic technique known as mindfulness has gained a great deal of attention. This approach is based on the Buddhist tradition but now is often a secular practice. Mindfulness is similar to meditation in the sense that it attempts to help us slow down and live in the moment and, in terms of therapy, this technique has been specifically adapted into a series of exercises that aim to reduce stress and the physiological manifestations of the stress response, known as Mindfulness Based Stress Reduction or MBSR. There are now innumerable books on the market that describe mindfulness techniques so we won't go into too much detail here as this approach hasn't been investigated a great deal with regard to the symptoms of the menopause. However there have been some initial promising findings.

Mindfulness-based stress reduction (MBSR) for menopausal symptoms

One small research study looked at 15 women who had a moderate or severe level of menopausal symptoms.[115] The women attended eight weekly MBSR classes within the University of Massachusetts Medical School. On average, the women reported a 40 per cent reduction in hot flushes four weeks following the end of the MBSR programme and they also said they felt better in terms of overall quality of life. The results from this study are evidently limited as the group was small and there was not a comparison group undergoing another type of therapy. However, due to the substantial amount of evidence that has shown this technique's ability to reduce stress,[116] we should see more research efforts dedicated to this area.

Relaxation training for menopausal symptoms

Various forms of relaxation training have garnered attention in terms of their ability to help with the management of menopausal symptoms. These include muscle relaxation, slowing down and pacing breathing patterns, and guided imagery. Overall these techniques appeared to reduce overall menopausal symptoms, vasomotor symptoms, and psychological symptoms such as mood.[117] However, some of the results from these studies were mixed showing no greater benefit than HRT (Chapter 7) or acupuncture (Chapter 5) so although you may want to introduce some relaxation techniques into your symptom management plan, this should be as an addition rather than substitute for a more effective treatment.

Take home message for other psychological therapies

▶ MBSR has been demonstrated consistently to reduce stress and early studies show promise in its ability to help with menopausal symptoms.

▶ Relaxation training and exercises may help with a range of menopausal symptoms within a comprehensive treatment plan.

How do I find a qualified therapist?

The first point of call for any adjunct therapy should be your GP or primary care practitioner. They will have registered and qualified therapists in your area and you might be able to get a direct referral which can cut the costs of therapy dramatically and/or be covered by health insurance. Also, many doctors and nurse practitioners are being trained in psychological therapies and larger doctors' practices may have on-site therapists. These can be fully trained and accredited psychologists (who will be qualified to doctoral level) or therapists specially trained in one technique such as CBT. Even if your doctor or specialist does not offer psychological therapy as part of their clinic, it is always advisable to tell her every additional approach you are using to tackle symptoms so that she has the complete picture of your healthcare plan.

However, you may want to find a therapist yourself so here is some advice on sourcing a reputable practitioner.

Cognitive behavioural therapists

As stated above, CBT is now a very common technique used in the West for a considerable number of conditions and symptoms. However, CBT training can vary a great deal and not all practitioners who say they are trained are qualified to a high standard. Accredited clinical and counselling psychologists will have completed education, training, and lengthy practice in this technique. The governing body in the UK for psychologists is the British Psychological Society (BPS) and only psychologists who have successfully fulfilled the BPS training programmes are eligible for 'chartered status'. This entails a minimum of six years of study and supervised sessions within validated institutions. These courses are competitive and so anyone who has achieved this status will no doubt be proficient in the types of psychological techniques they offer individuals. Psychologists also must maintain their skills via continuing professional development which is reviewed annually. Therefore, a chartered psychologist should be up-to-date in the latest methods and aware of research in their areas of expertise.

The BPS has a directory which can be searched by area and by technique (please see the Useful Addresses/Websites section at the end of this book for the web link). To search specifically for a qualified psychologist that offers CBT simply type in 'CBT' in the 'Additional Information' tab at the bottom of the page. You can also identify psychologists trained in mindfulness techniques in this way. Additionally, you can search for practitioners who specialise in certain types of problems under the 'What are the Issues?' section; there is not a drop-down option for menopausal symptoms but within the 'general health' menu, 'general health', 'stress management', and possibly 'sleeping disorders' may narrow down your search.

However, this is where searching for a therapist can seem rather confusing as the BPS directory list does not tell you if the professionals on the search list are 'practitioner psychologists'. A practitioner psychologist is someone who has trained purposely to deliver therapeutic techniques rather than work in academia or research for instance. But you can also check for this via the Health and Care Professions Council (HCPC; please see the Useful Addresses/Websites section) which regulates practitioner psychologists.

Like the BPS, the HCPC has certain standards and requirements that individuals must demonstrate to be able to use practitioner titles. These titles are protected by law so no one can advertise themselves as one of these protected titles unless they are registered with the HCPC. In addition to a number of psychologists such as a practitioner psychologist, clinical psychologist and counselling psychologist, there are other types of practitioners within the HCPC's remit that have protected titles: physiotherapists, dieticians, paramedics, and biomedical scientists, for example. So anyone using one of these labels correctly will have met strict criteria terms of professional skills, education, and behavioural practices which safeguard the public against harm. The HCPC has substantial power and can prevent an individual from practising if they do not meet the established standards and/or if a member of the public makes a complaint that is upheld. This is exactly the same as medical doctors where the General Medical Council (GMC) oversees clinical care and can withdraw a licence if necessary (this is covered more in Chapter 5 with regard to Complementary and Alternative Medicine (CAM) and its practitioners).

The HCPC site also has a searchable register (the Useful Addresses/Websites section contains the exact webpage for this) but you must know who you are looking for and search via their name or registration number. Hence, it is worth compiling a list of possible psychologists in your area from the BPS database and then checking whether they are currently registered with the HCPC if you want to make sure that your practitioner has undergone the most robust training and examination.

However, this does not mean that a therapist who is not entered into these databases cannot carry out CBT; there are just not such strict safeguards in place. Other professionals such as counsellors and psychotherapists may administer mixed approaches that have a CBT component. The British Association for Behavioural and Cognitive Psychotherapies (BABCP) also has a register which includes therapists that have completed an accredited CBT course (see Useful Addresses/Websites). As mentioned previously, other types of professionals do receive training in CBT such as medical doctors, social workers, and occupational therapists, and details of these individuals will be held on the BABCP register. You can either search by the person's surname if you want to check an individual's accreditation information or you can do a geographical search for accredited therapists in your area.

Hypnotherapists

Hypnotherapists are not as heavily regulated as practitioner psychologists but again, many different types of professional may have been trained in clinical hypnosis or hypnotherapeutic techniques. However, the title 'hypnotherapist' is not protected and the profession isn't regulated in the UK. This means that anyone can call themselves a 'hypnotherapist' with no formal or fairly minimal training in the technique (sometimes just a weekend-length course). Like CAM practitioners discussed in Chapter 5 there is no governing body that you can complain to if you're unhappy with a hypnotherapist's treatment, unless of course this person is also a doctor or psychologist and a member of another regulatory body. This can result in some inadequate practices with little recourse except if an individual has described themselves inaccurately within marketing material and then you may want to get in contact with the Advertising Standards Authority (ASA; see Useful Addresses/Websites), which has special guidelines for individuals and companies offering health and beauty advice and products. You can also search the ASA's site for previous rulings following on from complaints; for instance if you enter the term 'hypnotherapy' into the 'search rulings' bar a number of upheld complaints are listed in this field (see Useful Addresses/Websites). This does not necessarily mean that these groups have done anything wrong other than overstate their claims of efficacy and treatment effects; but these can be misleading and you have a right to know of limitations of a particular method. Trading Standards can also be contacted if you feel unhappy with a commercial treatment or product (see Useful Addresses/Websites).

However, there are a number of bodies which produce lists of practitioners, such as hypnotherapists, who adhere to their guidelines or standards. It should be noted that adherence is voluntary rather than statutory. There are numerous organisations that do this and you can research this further on the Hypnotherapy Directory website (see Useful Addresses/Websites). This site also allows you to search for a hypnotherapist who is a member of a professional body and this will give you a list of vetted therapists. Do bear in mind though that these bodies do not have the governing powers that organisations such as the GMC or BPS have, so here are a few questions that you can ask a potential therapist in order to find assess her approach and professionalism:

▶ How many people have you treated with menopausal symptoms?

▶ Can you please explain your hypnotherapy technique for menopausal symptoms?

▶ Do you have any information on average success rates/benefits/symptom reduction following your treatment? Was this information collected by you or an external organisation?

▶ How many sessions would you recommend? (The hypnotherapist may not be able to answer this until after an initial consultation.)

▶ What are the costs and cancellations policies? (In general, a hypnotherapy session usually costs between £50 and £90 but the first session may be more due to time taken to discuss and evaluate your symptoms. Most therapists would require a 24-hour notice of cancellation and may charge the full cost of the session or a percentage if cancellation is made in less than 24 hours.)

▶ Do you offer concessionary rates for people on low/ fixed incomes such as retired persons and those on benefits (if necessary)?

▶ Can I speak to someone with similar symptoms to mine who has been helped by you?

▶ What is your complaints policy/procedure? May I have a copy of this?

Remember you can speak to as many therapists as you like before opting for one particular individual. In general, we would advise that if anyone tries to give you the hard-sell or pressure you into booking straight away or block booking before you've had your first session you should consider looking elsewhere.

Chapter 4 summary

For women who may not be able to use HRT or medical interventions to control the symptoms of the menopause, or those that don't want to subject themselves to the risks and side effects of such treatments, psychological therapies are certainly an attractive option. We suggest that these types of techniques can be integrated into a wider treatment plan which could include, for instance, nutritional or dietary changes (Chapters 2 and 3), general health maintenance (Chapter 2), and self-help such as sleep hygiene practices (Chapter 6). You may also want to consider Complementary and Alternative Medicine (CAM) possibilities, which we will outline in the next chapter.

Chapter 5

COMPLEMENTARY AND ALTERNATIVE MEDICINE (CAM) THERAPIES

There are numerous Complementary and Alternative Medicine (CAM) techniques that have been used by women for many decades to help them manage and cope with the intrusive and at times distressing symptoms of the menopause. In this chapter we will explore the CAM therapies that have been studied and evaluated through academic and scientific research. Hence, this is not a comprehensive list of all the CAM techniques available – indeed the list is seemingly endless as novel methods are developed and marketed to women. Here we have chosen to include just the techniques that have an (at least) emerging evidence base to ensure that you have an objective view of the utility of CAM therapies. However, the depth and breadth of research will not be to the degree of HRT for various reasons, most often lack of funding (the very nature of CAM is that it is not something large pharmaceutical companies will invest in and governmental research funding is often hard to come by for non-orthodox techniques).

Mind–body medicine

All the therapies outlined in this chapter can be held under the banner of 'mind–body' medicine. You will undoubtedly be aware of this description and have most likely tried some of these techniques throughout your life. Indeed, a wealth of research now supports these methods for various long-term conditions and also stress reduction and energy optimisation. We are becoming increasingly aware of the mechanisms by which these types of therapies work, in addition to determining their effectiveness; in other words, some methods that might have previously been considered as unscientific are gaining credibility. But there is still some way to go with regard to being able to draw clear conclusions about the efficacy of CAM techniques for menopausal symptoms. Nevertheless, unlike traditional HRT, CAM methods are low risk in terms of side effects and potential harms to patients, so many women choose to explore these types of treatments, either as a substitute for HRT or as an adjunct therapy.

Use of CAM by women

A large proportion of women experiencing perimenopause, menopause or postmenopausal symptoms make use of CAM techniques; research studies suggest between 40 and 76 per cent of women have tried at least one CAM option.[118,119] The most commonly used techniques appear to be relaxation and stress management[120] (as discussed in the previous chapter), diet/nutrition, exercise such as yoga[121] and herbal medicine.[122]

But of course there are many other types of CAM methods that women seek out to help with the symptoms of menopause and also general wellbeing. For example, one Australian study found that the most frequently consulted practitioners were naturopaths and acupuncturists; although chiropractic treatment and massage were reported as the most effective methods for symptom reduction, in addition to nutrition.[123] There are also numerous over-the-counter preparations including evening primrose oil and black cohosh tablets (as outlined in Chapter 3), which nearly 60 per cent of women in the aforementioned Australian study used at some point.[124]

In the USA, older women, those with a higher level of education and whose health was poor were more likely to try CAM[125] and in the UK, women from a White ethnic background, who were physically active and did not smoke were more likely to use CAM than others.[126]

Reasons to use CAM

Simply knowing the demographic characteristics of women doesn't tell us a great deal about why they chose to add CAM into their treatment programmes or lifestyle changes. You will have your own individual and unique reasons for all your choices regarding treatment but it can be interesting to know why other women have opted for these methods as some traditional (orthodox) doctors have been rather dismissive of these techniques due to their lack of evidence. An enlightening study which interviewed 44 women, both CAM and non-CAM users, found that one primary reason for going down the CAM route was the belief that these techniques were more 'natural' than HRT.[127] However, the exact meaning of the word 'natural' varied greatly between the women; for some it denoted the belief that CAM was safer than orthodox medications, for others it portrayed the notion that the menopause in itself was a natural process in life rather than a disease and as such anything used to help with symptoms should also be 'natural'. Other women in this study mentioned that their mothers and grandmothers didn't use medicines or concern their doctors with the menopause and so they wanted to avoid that approach also. Some of the interviewees also said that CAM techniques often claim to redress balance in the body, and so appeared to be more natural than traditional medicine. Most of the women had more than one idea about what constituted 'natural' which is perhaps unsurprising in the context of complex decisions regarding healthcare.

Another interesting finding in this study was that the women who used CAM methods had often had success in the past with CAM for other ailments or symptoms not associated with the menopause. Some of these women opted for CAM as a first choice when experiencing symptoms, although others only sought out CAM treatments when orthodox medicine failed to alleviate the complaint. This may be why older women and those who had poorer health have been found to be more likely to use CAM, i.e. simply because they had more opportunities to do so before the onset of menopause, hence had more positive encounters with these techniques and practitioners.

One final notable finding of the Hill-Sakurai *et al.* (2008) study was that, in comparison to the CAM users, the non-CAM users felt the notion of 'natural' was outdated and unscientific and their discussion of the menopause was more in terms of biology than life stages.[128] Regardless of others' views on CAM, we hope the following information sheds some light on whether one, or more, of these methods may be right for you.

Yoga

As noted, yoga is one of the most commonly used types of CAM by women experiencing the menopause. Yoga stems from ancient Indian philosophy and although historically this practice was associated with Hinduism and Buddhism, in modern times it can be explored as a secular method to increase health and wellbeing. There are numerous types of yoga (e.g. Hatha, Iyengar, Viniyoga, Sivananda, etc.) but in its most basic form it is a combination of stretching poses and controlled breathing techniques. Often, however, yoga classes also include narrative on uniting the mind, body, and spirit. In the West, yoga is generally taught as a series of physical postures (asana), breathing techniques (pranayama), and meditation (dyana).

Research has been conducted on the benefits of yoga for numerous conditions and health complaints, including chronic pain, fatigue, psychological distress, high blood pressure, body weight, cholesterol, and elevated glucose levels.[129,130] There have also been a number of studies that have looked at whether yoga can help menopausal women; recently groups of researchers have looked at this evidence as a whole in order to come to a conclusion not only on whether yoga is useful in this context, but also on what symptoms or aspects of the menopause it helps with most.

One review by a group in Germany identified five high-quality studies that compared yoga to another type of exercise or no treatment.[131] Across these five studies a total of 582 women took part in the interventions. The researchers looked at comparisons of different types of symptoms such as depression, anxiety, and sleep problems (psychological symptoms); pain and fatigue (somatic symptoms); hot flushes and night sweats (vasomotor symptoms); and sexual dysfunctions and bladder problems (urogenital symptoms). Overall, when the studies were pooled, there was some evidence for short-term improvements in the symptoms characterised as psychological. But when the studies were taken together, rather than individual findings, there was not strong evidence for the benefits of yoga for overall menopausal symptoms or any of the other symptom categories.

Therefore, what can we conclude about the usefulness of yoga for perimenopausal and menopausal women? Sleep disturbance, anxiety, and low mood are common and at times distressing and intrusive symptoms, not just of menopause but of many, many conditions and in themselves. As we age, other health issues may rear their head such as high blood pressure and high cholesterol levels and it can become increasingly difficult to maintain a healthy weight. Yoga has been shown to be a useful tool in managing these concerns, so you may want to try a beginners or intermediate class if you've never practised yoga before. Hatha yoga may be a good place to start as it is one of the most frequently offered types of yoga in Western countries and it is suggested for beginners/intermediate level. Very vigorous yoga (i.e. 'dynamic' yoga) and 'hot' yoga classes are not normally recommended for women experiencing symptoms such as hot flushes, fatigue, and other symptoms associated with the menopause.

Take home message for yoga

▶ Yoga can help to improve general wellbeing, anxiety, depression, and poor sleep during the menopause.

▶ Yoga can also aid weight control and reduce high blood pressure and cholesterol, which are health concerns that can affect women later in life.

Acupuncture

Acupuncture is a technique that originated in ancient China and is based on a holistic view of the body and health and illness. Acupuncture aims to restore balance within the body by stimulating particular acupuncture points, of which there are 365 in total, lying along 20 'meridians'. Energy or 'Qi' flows along these meridians, and acupuncture theory states that if there is a blockage in the flow of Qi from one meridian to another, symptoms, illness, or disease will exist.[132]

Acupuncture can be administrated by placing needles on the acupuncture points, pressure (known as acupressure), or via electrical stimulation (electro-acupuncture). Acupuncture is a widely used treatment throughout the world for numerous health complaints and illnesses, including respiratory disorders such as allergic rhinitis, premenstrual syndrome, hypotension, and depression but most notably in chronic pain where its effects have been demonstrated as comparable to morphine.[133] In fact, the World Health Organisation supports the use of acupuncture in 43 diseases.

The physiological explanation for these findings has attracted a good deal of attention. Indeed, as the pain relieving impact of acupuncture has been shown time and time again, it has been labelled 'acupuncture analgesia'. Acupuncture analgesia appears to occur via numerous neuronal pathways and genetic differences in physiology also appear to be important with regard to treatment effects.[134] This level of detail is perhaps unnecessary when considering whether to try acupuncture for the symptoms of the menopause; suffice to say that the underlying reasons for the benefits of acupuncture have been explored by many researchers using various methodologies including brain imaging and the evidence is quite convincing for its utility in pain relief at least.[135]

In terms of specific menopausal symptoms, there is mixed evidence for the benefits of acupuncture. By pooling 16 studies, with 1155 women, the authors of a review on the effectiveness of acupuncture for hot flushes concluded that the evidence was insufficient to support the use of acupuncture for this symptom.[136] However, in a review of 12 studies, totalling 869 women, the long-term effects of acupuncture on hot flushes was shown to be promising, reducing the occurrence and severity of this symptom.[137] Psychological, somatic, and urogenital symptoms also improved across these studies. However, when digging a bit deeper into this research, it seems that acupuncture may be no better than 'sham acupuncture'. This is a technique used in research studies which mimics acupuncture but is not 'real' acupuncture; for instance a practitioner may insert the needles into points on the body that aren't traditional acupuncture points. But in both reviews women who underwent acupuncture had better outcomes than those who had no treatment. Nevertheless, overall acupuncture appeared less effective than HRT.

Take home message for acupuncture

▸ If you're worried about the side effects of HRT, acupuncture is better for the symptoms of menopause than no treatment at all.

▸ If you experience pain, either in conjunction with other menopause symptoms or as a result of another illness, there is good evidence to embark on a series of acupuncture treatments with a qualified acupuncturist.

Reflexology

Reflexology has some similarities to acupuncture as the rationale for this technique is that there are certain areas of the foot and hand that correspond to organs, glands, and other bodily parts and that by stimulating these points, health benefits will occur in the corresponding body part. The historical background of reflexology is unclear; however is does seem that Ancient Egyptians used reflexology, or at least a form of foot massage for health and wellbeing.[138] Also, there is some mention of reflexology as an ancient Indian and Chinese technique, in conjunction with acupuncture.[139]

Modern-day reflexology practitioners consider the mechanism by which this therapy works is through the regaining of balance and homeostasis which will, in turn, allow the body to heal itself. The more precise theories regarding physiological pathways to explain any treatment benefits are improvements in blood flow, activation of the parasympathetic nervous system, and enhancement of nerve connections in the body.[140,141,142] However, none of these theories have been supported adequately through scientific research at this point and reflexologists often cite other factors such as the release of endorphins and the general impact of seeing a compassionate therapist.

There is less published research on the benefits of reflexology for menopausal symptoms than other CAM methods but there have been some trials. One research group from the School of Complementary Health in Exeter, UK compared reflexology to non-specific foot massage. Seventy-six women had six weekly treatments, followed by a further three monthly sessions, hence nine treatments in total over four to five months. The researchers measured the women's rating of menopausal symptoms and psychological symptoms such as anxiety and depression. Although the self-reported ratings of anxiety and depression improved after treatment, and the frequency and severity of hot flushes and night sweats also decreased, this happened in both groups. In other words, reflexology was not better for treating psychological and menopausal symptoms than a general foot massage in this study.[143]

However, when looking at reviews of reflexology, this technique does appear to offer some health benefits for other conditions such as diabetes, premenstrual syndrome, cancer, multiple sclerosis, and dementia.[144] But the authors of this review did note that the evidence wasn't of a high enough quality to be able to state with certainty that reflexology is an effective treatment for any condition or set of symptoms.

Nevertheless, if you are experiencing sleep difficulties, reflexology may be advantageous to you as demonstrated in a study by Asltoghiri and Ghodsi (2012).[145] Here, the percentage of menopausal woman who also had a sleep disorder decreased following 21 days of brief treatment (lasting only 15 minutes) of either reflexology or non-specific foot massage. Unlike the Williamson *et al.* (2002) study,[146] the reflexology treatment was superior to the general foot massage as 41.5 per cent of women reported normal sleep after therapy, compared to only 19.1 per cent in the massage group.

Take home message for reflexology

▶ Reflexology does not appear to help with either psychological or specific menopausal symptoms.

▶ Reflexology shows more promise to help with sleep disturbance in women experiencing the menopause.

Other CAM methods

As mentioned in the introduction, there is a raft of CAM therapies that women have tried in order to reduce the symptoms of the menopause. The techniques outlined above have the most evidence for our consideration but others have also been researched, albeit not as comprehensively. However, the following treatments are worth a mention, either due to their lack of support from the scientific community, or because they have been studied with regard to a specific symptom.

Homeopathy

Homeopathy is a form of treatment that uses very diluted substances (in the homeopathic school of thought, the more a substance is diluted, the greater its healing properties) that are also subject to a series of shaking; taken together these processes are called succession. This concept was first proposed by the German doctor Samuel Hahnemann in 1796, who developed homeopathy on the notion 'may like be cured by like'.[147] However, in 2010 a House of Commons Science and Technology Committee report stated that the underpinnings of this technique were scientifically implausible (i.e. diluting and shaking a substance cannot turn it into a medicine) and that there was no evidence that homeopathy can effectively treat any condition.[148] Yet, many people choose this method; in 2007 nearly five million American adults and children sought advice from homeopaths.[149]

As homeopaths create personalised care plans for patients, there are no set protocols for menopause; however the most commonly used preparations for menopausal symptoms are Lachesis (formulated from the South American Bushmaster snake venom), Pulsatilla (formulated from the Anemone pulsatilla, a perennial windflower), and Sepia (formulated from cuttlefish ink).[150] A clinical audit of a community menopause clinic in Sheffield, UK reported improvements in a range of symptoms including headaches, hot flushes, fatigue, and psychological symptoms following one consultation per month for six months with a homeopath and personalised homeopathic medicines.[151] However, as there was no comparison group in this study (because it was simply an audit of an existing service, rather than a research study *per se*), it's not possible to say if the benefits were directly due to the homeopathic remedies or whether the therapeutic gains were solely from interacting with the homeopaths; or even if people would have improved over time with no treatment. Indeed, a review of the research on homeopathy for menopausal symptoms concluded it was unclear whether the benefits seen across a range of studies could truly be afforded to the homeopathic preparations.[152] Rather, it might be that the entire homeopathic 'package', which includes in-depth consultations by an empathic practitioner, leads to changes in symptoms and how these are viewed. In this analysis it could be said that homeopathy had a positive, but placebo, effect on women undergoing the menopause. Further research may give us more clues as to whether homeopathic remedies work in the manner by which has been described. At present, many scientists and doctors are sceptical about this technique, most notably because after the process of succession, it is improbable any of the original substance will remain in the remedy. In other words, homeopathic preparations are likely to be no more than small bottles of water.

Take home message for homeopathy

▸ There is not sufficient evidence to support the mechanisms of action for homeopathy or its effects on menopausal symptoms.

Tai chi

Tai chi is another ancient Chinese practice that has been used for many centuries for health and wellbeing, although it is also a form of martial art. Like yoga, tai chi integrates breathing techniques with 'exercise', but in this method the deep breathing techniques are coupled with slow, controlled movements.[153] Also like yoga, there are now many different forms of tai chi, the most popular and readily available being yang, wu, and tai chi chih (however, unless you visit a specialist centre, you'll most likely be offered 'tai chi', not a specific form).

Tai chi has been found to improve quality of life, diminish anxiety and depression, limit falls in older adults, maintain heart health, and enhance general physical functioning.[154] In terms of the menopause, tai chi has been investigated in relation to osteoporosis in postmenopausal women. In a study of 132 postmenopausal women (but within ten years of menopause onset) bone mineral density was compared between women who practised tai chi for 45 minutes, five days a week and those that had a more sedentary lifestyle. After one year, both the women using tai chi and the sedentary women demonstrated bone loss, however the rate of loss was slower (2.6- to 3.6-fold deceleration) in those that practiced tai chi.[155] Additionally, only one woman who used tai chi suffered a fracture over the year's observation whereas three women who did not use this form of physical activity experienced a fracture.

However, as is so often the case with research, further studies did not support the benefits of tai chi for maintaining bone mineral density in postmenopausal woman, either in comparison to other forms of exercise or calcium supplements.[156]

Take home message for tai chi

▶ Tai chi is better for preventing osteoporosis than doing no exercise at all, but does not appear to be superior to general forms of physical activity or calcium supplements.

How to find a reputable CAM therapist

Now that you have reviewed the evidence for a range of CAM therapies, you may want to seek out a therapist. Here we offer some advice on the best way to find a qualified and reputable CAM practitioner; it is mainly common sense but when we are experiencing a myriad of symptoms and in serious need of relief, it can be beneficial just to remind ourselves of a few golden rules. There are many excellent therapists out there, so don't let any of the below hinder you from seeking the care of a CAM professional. However, CAM is not subject to statutory professional regulation in the same way that conventional medicine is. This means there are not laws in place that ensure that CAM practitioners are adequately qualified/trained and monitored to ensure they adhere to standard codes of practice, as there are for doctors. In other words, you are less protected as a patient when you visit a CAM therapist as opposed to a medical doctor. Osteopaths and chiropractors are regulated in the same way as medics and are now not considered to be CAM practitioners although they once were. As they are regulated, these professionals must follow strict guidelines and be subject to robust scrutiny throughout their careers. This is of course not to say that other kinds of CAM practitioners do not observe high standards, they are just not legally compelled to do so.

Medical doctors are regulated by the General Medical Council (GMC), which checks the qualifications of doctors, monitors their practice and will investigate any complaints made against medics and take appropriate action (the same applies for the General Osteopathic Council and the General Chiropractic Council). This type of organisation does not exist for CAM but there are bodies that CAM practitioners can register with that have systems of checking qualifications and ensuring continuing professional development. For instance, the Complementary and Natural Healthcare Council (CNHC) is a voluntary register for a number of practitioners working in the CAM field including yoga therapists, acupuncturists, reflexologists, and nutritional therapists, amongst others. The CNHC has a Code of Conduct, Ethics and Performance that practitioners need to adhere to and practitioners must also have the correct education, training, and qualifications in order to be included on the CNHC register. This register is approved by the Professional Standards Authority for Health and Social Care, which is the same organisation that oversees the GMC. Therefore, those who are listed on the CNHC register will need to have met a high level of training and professional development so there is a degree of assurance in the skills of CAM practitioners on this directory.

Nevertheless, it is worth bearing in mind that anyone can set themselves up as a CAM therapist, whether they have been trained or not, or with minimal training. It is not illegal to do this and therefore if you consult with such a practitioner and you're unsatisfied or have been made unwell then there is very little recourse for you besides your usual civil rights. Hence, it is up to you to do some research on your CAM practitioner and decide if you feel comfortable with them and their approach. Here are a few tips to help you with this decision:

▶ Ask if the practitioner is a member of any professional bodies, bearing in mind these are limited in their scope and do not have the same powers as a statutory professional regulatory body. Nevertheless, checks are carried out by the organisations noted above which ensure that the therapists have relevant training.

▶ If the practitioner is not a member of a regulatory body at all, you may want to check their qualifications (in fact, it is a good idea to do this regardless of organisation membership). But a long list of letters after a name doesn't necessarily mean that the individual has studied for decades in their chosen field. Some qualifications can be as little as a weekend course. You should be able to find out what any abbreviations mean by a simple internet search or asking the practitioner directly. If they are reluctant to discuss this with you then we would suggest looking elsewhere for a CAM therapist.

▶ Many practitioners, not just CAM therapists, use testimonials on their websites. Whilst these may appear to be impressive, they should not be considered as 'evidence' or proof of effectiveness. You may want to ask any prospective practitioners if they have research evidence for their practice. As we have seen in this chapter, studies can be contradictory and conclusions difficult to draw so it would be unlikely that a CAM therapist would be able to show you a wealth of positive study findings. Rather, our advice is to opt for a practitioner who is honest about the current evidence base and recognises that more work needs to be done to support claims of efficacy in their chosen field.

▶ Similar to the point above, if a practitioner or CAM/ holistic/integrative clinic has information on client satisfaction, bear in mind that yet again this is not 'proof' that the technique will help you with the symptoms of the menopause. Most of us feel better after speaking to a practitioner that has the time to listen to us properly, and this in itself can act as a soothing balm. But to be able to state the usefulness of a particular therapy, there would need to be a comparison group to ensure that any effects or improvements were due to the therapy alone and not something else such as a good bedside manner (although we are not trivialising the importance of the latter). Also, any research should be conducted by independent organisations, not the practitioners or clinics themselves, to remove bias.

▶ CAM can be expensive; very few modalities are covered on the NHS and only some within health insurances policies so you may want to query the number of sessions a practitioner recommends before you start the treatment. Be wary of two-for-one offers or deals on coupons sites however.

If you feel happy that you have been given enough information about the technique of choice, then do give it a go. Please also tell your GP or specialist what additional methods you are trying so that they have the entire picture regarding your symptom management strategy. A recent study illustrated that numerous women embark on CAM within gaining advice from a CAM practitioner or their doctor.[157] The authors of this study urged primary care doctors to be more familiar with current research on CAM techniques for the symptoms of the menopause so that they can provide safe, effective, and co-ordinated care to their patients. Even if your doctor is dismissive or lacks knowledge of CAM therapies, it's better that they know what help you're seeking and methods you're trying as certain herbs, for instance, can interact with drugs.

Chapter 5 summary

In this chapter we've outlined a number of CAM therapies but these are by no means the only techniques on offer in the alternative healthcare market. We focused on the modalities that have been researched in the greatest detail, so that we can be confident in our recommendations to you. This does not mean that other techniques are not beneficial for perimenopausal or menopausal women; research is continually conducted and in time other treatments may be shown to reduce the symptoms associated with the menopause. But for now, our suggestions are cautious. Nevertheless, this chapter has illustrated that whilst CAM techniques can help with some psychological symptoms such as anxiety and depression and also sleep disturbance, to date there is limited evidence that they can effectively treat other menopause-related complaints. But it must be noted that many of the studies carried out by researchers have only looked at hot flushes and one other menopause-related symptom, not the full range of symptoms experienced. As noted by Woods *et al.*,[158] it's important that future researchers look at the full scope of symptoms so that we can evaluate more precisely which CAM techniques help which aspects of the menopause. This will allow medics and practitioners to integrate CAM modalities and orthodox medicine into a personalised treatment plan for women experiencing the menopause. In addition, many CAM techniques have been shown to benefit issues such as heart disease and osteoporosis, which of course are concerns for menopausal and postmenopausal women; i.e. you may want to use CAM for reasons other than specific symptoms associated with the menopause.

In the next chapter we will look at some self-help techniques that can help you cope with menopausal symptoms and also improve quality of life.

Chapter 6

SELF-HELP

In this chapter, we will outline some more general techniques you can use on a day-to-day basis to deal with specific symptoms, relationship difficulties, and the more general feelings of lethargy and low mood. Menopausal and postmenopausal years can, and should, be one of the most enjoyable phases in a women's life; as child-rearing, domestic and sometimes work responsibilities wind down, careers, hobbies, and leisure activities can have a major boost. By controlling unpleasant symptoms during the menopause, these needn't be 'lost' years; but rather life can be taken by the horns and personal growth and transformation can occur. Nevertheless, we will start in this chapter by looking at how to spot symptom triggers and how these can be avoided or dealt with.

Identifying symptom triggers

Although there are some foods, drinks, and situations that seem to elicit particular symptoms in women during the menopause, no two women will have the same triggers or the same set of symptoms. Therefore, it's advisable to take a methodological approach to identifying symptom triggers, rather than using guesswork. We suggest using a symptom diary of which there are many versions. You can either download a diary from the internet, use a smartphone app, or simply try a 'pen and paper' method that works just as well as a more technological approach (see Table 6.1).

Using a symptom diary

To construct a symptom diary, follow the steps below:

▶ Draw a grid with the time of day in the first column. Make sure to jot down the date too as there may be a weekly pattern to symptom occurrence.

▶ The next column will record your symptoms. Note down all the symptoms you experience including emotional and cognitive types of symptoms (e.g. feeling irritable or tearful, depression, anxiety, problems concentrating, poor memory, etc.).

▶ The severity of the symptom should be recorded also on a scale of 1–10, with 10 reflecting a symptom being 'as bad as it could be'. Here, the length of the symptom should also be noted if relevant; for instance you can log the length of a hot flush or headache but dry skin and muscle aches are harder to quantify in a daily diary.

▶ Next, and this is important when considering the discussion later in this chapter on the interpretation of symptoms, enter the influence the symptom has had on your normal activities, with 1 equalling 'no impact at all' and 10 meaning 'I have not been able to carry out my usual activities due to this symptom'.

▶ Food and drink consumed in the day should also be included in the symptom diary. Although alcohol, caffeine, and spicy food can trigger certain menopausal symptoms such as hot flushes and headaches, other foods and beverages can be culprits for different women.

▶ In terms of the column labelled 'feelings and stressors', these can be general feelings (both good and bad although the latter are more likely to act as a trigger) and situations that cause you to feel anxious or stressed. Examples include one-off events such as giving a presentation at work, weekly demands like looking after elderly parents, or a low-level and overall sense of 'just not feeling right/like myself' should be logged.

▶ Finally include any techniques you are using to deal with your symptoms currently. This can be over-the-counter medication such as pain relief, psychological strategies as discussed in Chapter 4, or something more practical like turning the thermostat down in your house when you've had a hot flush.

▶ If you're having night-time symptoms they can be recorded in the morning as we wouldn't advise getting up and jotting these down at the time as this may make it harder to get back to sleep.

▶ You may want to complete a weekly diary instead of a daily grid if your symptoms are less frequent.

TABLE 6.1 SYMPTOM AND FOOD DIARY TO HELP IDENTIFY SYMPTOM PATTERNS AND TRIGGERS

Event time	Symptom type	Severity (1–10); length	Impact (1–10)	Food / drink consumed	Feelings and stressors	Strategies used
Night symptoms	Night sweats	7; think I was sweating for a few hours before I couldn't stand it anymore	8 –; couldn't get back to sleep		Felt fed up	Had to change clothes in the night
Wake time: 7.02					Woke up feeling dreadful; another bad night and stressed about the day ahead	Tried to practise mindfulness after waking; finding it tricky
7.28				Large coffee w. milk and 2 x sugars		
7.43	Headache	6; lasted 45 mins			I know I shouldn't drink coffee on an empty stomach	Paracetomol 2 x 500g
7.47				Quick bowl of cereal	Berated myself for not eating	
11.02	Hot flush	4 mins	9		So embarrassing as was in meeting	Deep breathing exercise quietly to myself

cont.

TABLE 6.1 [CONT.]

Event time	Symptom type	Severity (1–10); length	Impact (1–10)	Food / drink consumed	Feelings and stressors	Strategies used
12.55				Chicken pesto pasta salad, snack crackers, fizzy apple juice		
13.14	Tearful				Felt stupidly upset by comment from a colleague	Told myself it wasn't personal (need more practice at this...)
15.03	Mid-aft dip as always; can't concentrate			Fruit salad		Wanted coffee, had fruit instead
18.30					Feel much better in myself; think it's more to do with chatting to other women at class than anything else	Rejuvenating yoga class
20.11				Starving so had chicken pie, veg and mash	Nice that hubby made me dinner	
etc.						
Sleep time: 00.33						

Diaries can also be used to track changes in menstruation during perimenopause in the form of a menstrual period diary. To use one of these, record the start and end of your period, flow levels to see if menstruation is getting lighter (or heavier) and any irregularities such as spotting.

You can use the information from your diary to see any daily, weekly, or monthly symptom patterns, food and drinks to possibly avoid and to identify emotional and situational triggers so that these can be dealt with (by using some of the strategies in Chapters 2 and 4 and later in this chapter perhaps). You may also want to show your completed symptom diary to your doctor or healthcare practitioner. This in-depth data will help your doctor immensely when devising a treatment programme and appropriate support for you.

Managing your weight

Weight gain during the menopause can be particularly troublesome and distressing. Not only do sex hormones play a role in regulating appetite, the psychological symptoms that can arise during the menopause can lead women to turn to food as comfort. Whilst HRT can help counteract weight gain,[159] if you do not want to use HRT there are other ways to manage your weight now and throughout life, as detailed below:

▶ Avoid quick-fixes and crash diets. Not only are these unlikely to result in weight loss in the long term, they will also leave you deficient in important nutrients and minerals. See Chapters 2 and 3 for detailed guidance on nutrition and appropriate supplements during the menopause. Please note however that taking supplements should never be used in place of food.

▶ Similarly, foods marketed as 'low-fat' or 'no-fat' are not the solution that they are marketed as. To make up for the loss of flavour, these products often have high levels of salt and sugar and can contain more calories than original versions of certain foods. Rather than buying manipulated low-fat products, eat only a small amount of high-fat foods that you enjoy.

▶ Diet drinks also do not now appear to meet their claims. Consumption of such beverages are linked to obesity; in one large-scale study people who regularly drank diet soft drinks had a 47 per cent higher body mass index (BMI) than people who did not consume artificially enhanced colas and other beverages.[160] This appears to be because such drinks disrupt the reward centres in our brains.[161] Therefore, as with low-fat foods, if you genuinely enjoy fizzy drinks then have the occasional bottle of non-diet drink rather than turning to diet soft drinks in the mistaken belief that their low calorie content will aid weight loss.

▶ Identify comfort eating. Food can act as a great comfort so look closely at your symptom diary and see if you seem to be eating at times of anxiety or mood swings. People often eat out of sheer boredom so be vigilant to see if you turn to food when your mind wanders. If you think you eat due to either emotional reasons or out of boredom, it would be worth engaging in 'mindful eating'. This is a form of mindfulness that has been shown to help people limit their high-calorie food intake[162] and serving size.[163] To eat mindfully, try not to have meals and snacks when you're doing other things like working or watching TV; instead focus on the food, the feel of it in your mouth and the individual taste of each bite. For more on mindfulness, refer to Chapter 4.

▶ Try not to skip breakfast. Eating regular meals has important consequences for energy regulation and metabolism and has been related to reduced risk of obesity and long-term illness.[164] Skipping breakfast may seem like an easy way to limit calories but research has shown that it often leads people to consume more food later in the day with the result of higher calorific intake overall.[165]

▶ Have a little of what you fancy. As mentioned above crash diets rarely work long-term and are unhealthy so do have some chocolate or crisps occasionally if you enjoy them. Denying yourself small treats will not only make it less likely that you'll stick to a sensible eating plan, but also it's miserable to never have your favourite foods. This in itself can paradoxically lead to comfort eating and weight gain.

▶ Finally, follow general advice on eating enough fruit and vegetables each day and reduce processed and pre-packaged foods. This is of course difficult when we're busy and need a quick meal but keep in mind that eating well should help with energy levels; hence by investing time in healthy food, you may be able to buy back the time spent preparing and cooking it in terms of increased energy levels.

What's the best type of exercise during the menopause?

We all know how important it is to keep active throughout life and exercise is particularly important as women get older due the associated health problems that can develop once hormone levels change (as discussed in Chapter 1). We covered some forms of mind–body exercise in the previous chapter, including yoga and tai chi, and saw how research studies mainly demonstrated that doing any form of activity was beneficial to women during the menopause. If we consider specifically the issue of osteoporosis, there has been a great deal of research looking into different forms of exercise and how these can help to prevent bone loss and fractures. Women who exercise typically are 4 per cent less likely to suffer from a fracture than sedentary women and when using a combination exercise programme (which includes both aerobic exercise and strength building techniques), active women will experience 3.2 per cent less bone loss than those who do not exercise.[166] These figures may not seem particularly impressive but exercise also helps to reduce the risk of cardiovascular disease (CVD) in women regardless of whether the activity is gentle or vigorous.[167] It doesn't matter how old you are when you start exercising, being physically active will improve heart health irrespective of age; conversely prolonged sitting has been shown to increase the risk of CVD in women of all ages, ethnic groups and BMIs.[168] BMI is an important factor when considering risk of breast cancer in postmenopausal women as those with a high BMI (without family history of breast cancer) benefit particularly from exercise in reducing their risk of this form of cancer.[169]

Hence, exercise can help not only with general fitness and mood but it can also reduce the risk of experiencing the health problems that can come with menopausal hormone changes. The key in terms of exercise is to find something you particularly enjoy that raises your heart rate and also forces your bones to support the weight of your body. The simplest form of this type of exercise is walking which is good news as we also know that spending time outdoors increases our sense of wellbeing and has the added benefit of helping us maintain adequate levels of vitamin D (which also conserves bone health). Therefore, you don't need to buy any expensive fitness equipment, join a gym or commit to scheduled classes to exercise – simply go for a brisk walk most days and you'll be helping your body in so many ways.

Getting sufficient sleep

Poor sleep can be a truly exasperating aspect of the menopause. You may have always had trouble sleeping or you might have previously enjoyed sound sleep that is now disturbed by night sweats, for example.

General sleep hygiene

There are a number of general strategies that can be incorporated into your night time routine that are known to improve sleep quality. These 'sleep hygiene' recommendations are for everyone: men and women at all stages of life.

▶ The amount of sleep each of us requires is individual, although most people need around seven to nine hours per night. Although patterns of sleep may change as we age, sleep quality doesn't necessarily decline as we get older. Rather, health conditions such as heart disease and depression can affect our ability to get a good night's sleep.[170] Therefore, if you are having significant sleep difficulties and have tried the recommendations in this section to no avail, do see your doctor so that they can exclude other conditions that might have contributed to poor and unrefreshing sleep.

▶ Banish devices. The light from televisions, computers, tablets, and smartphones has been shown to disturb sleep in people of all ages.[171,172] Hence, the old adage that the bedroom should only be used for 'sleep and sex' is increasingly supported by research. Remove any

TVs and laptops from the bedroom and also leave the smartphones and tablets in other rooms of the house before bed. If you use your phone for an alarm clock don't use this as an excuse; invest in a simple bedside clock and don't check your email in the middle of the night. Even if you feel that games on your smartphone help you to unwind, the artificial light emitted can disrupt your natural circadian rhythm so it's best not to play these for at least an hour before going to bed. Similarly the light from e-readers negatively affects sleep quality therefore switch back to traditional paperback books at bedtime.[173]

▶ Other forms of light can also play havoc with your sleep. If you live in an area with a great deal of streetlight then blackout curtains and blinds can help. Also, the sun in the summer months can prompt wakefulness earlier than our natural wake time; hence ensuring your bedroom is dark enough for you at night can help you to drop off more easily and stay asleep longer.

▶ Noise can also prevent sleep initiation and promote wakefulness. If you live in a noisy area there are sound machines that can be purchased online and from larger chemists. They usually have settings of natural sounds like rainfall and ocean waves but you can also find white noise machines that emit a low, regular hum (think of the sound that used to be produced when a TV channel ceased transmission at night). Fans too can act as a type of noise machine as the continuous whirr will block out a good deal of external noise. You might want to invest in a fan to regulate your body temperature, as discussed in the section below.

▶ Food and drink can also influence how well we sleep. Although it's common knowledge that caffeine increases alertness, and so impedes sleep, it may be surprising to learn that some decaffeinated types of tea and coffee contain caffeine, albeit at much reduced levels. Check the ingredient lists to see how much caffeine remains in these products but you might want to opt for naturally decaffeinated hot drinks such as peppermint and herbal teas. Remember also that foods containing chocolate contain caffeine.

▶ Try to avoiding eating large meals, high-impact exercise, work and smoking in the evening (although smoking should be avoided at all times to limit menopausal symptoms). Whilst exercise is beneficial for overall health and to reduce the risk of menopause-related conditions such as heart disease and osteoporosis (Chapter 1), gentle and stress relieving exercise such as yoga and tai chi are better in the evening compared to vigorous activities such as running, Zumba and spin cycling.

▶ Although alcohol can make us feel sleepy, it does not result in restorative sleep. Alcohol reduces the amount of rapid eye movement (REM) stage sleep, so even though the hours may have ticked by and sleep has come to pass, it won't have the refreshing quality of natural sleep.[174] Also, even if you have a few glasses of wine to help you drop off at night, you're very likely to wake up later as your body metabolises the alcohol. The effects of alcohol on sleep quality can even occur following lunchtime drinking.

▶ The general belief about daytime napping is that it results in poor sleep. However, in a review of long and short naps and no napping, sleeping during the day didn't seem to have an effect on either the quality or quantity of night time sleep.[175] However, excessive daytime sleepiness can be a sign of serious conditions such as cardiovascular disease and Type 2 diabetes so if you do feel that you can't stay awake during the day, tell your doctor.

Sleep and the menopause

Symptoms specific to the menopause can make sleep very difficult also. Night sweats are a common symptom for many women both during and postmenopause. Hot flushes can also affect sleep quality and quantity so you may find that your sleep improves when these other symptoms are ameliorated. Nevertheless, here is some tailored advice for improving the nature of your sleep during the menopause:

▶ Maintaining a comfortable room temperature is advice given in both general sleep hygiene guidance and also as a way to combat hot flushes at night. This can be tricky if you and your partner differ in body temperature. First do try and openly discuss your needs with your spouse and come to a compromise. Perhaps introduce a fan in the bedroom that's only directed at you? Or ask your partner to wear more layers at night. A cool room aids sleep for most people so even if your other half is resistant to decreasing the temperature in the bedroom at first, ask him or her to try it to for a few nights and see if s/he can tolerate the cooler room.

▶ Wicking pyjamas are made from material that absorbs moisture and wicks it away so that nightclothes don't become drenched, leading to discomfort and shivering when experiencing night sweats. There are now many brands of wicking pyjamas and night gowns on the market which can easily be bought from online retailers.

▶ Women often report improved sleep quality when using HRT as menopausal symptoms decrease.[176] If you are using HRT, micronised progesterone (bioidentical – see Chapters 7 and 8) appears to benefit sleep more than medroxyprogesterone acetate (non-bioidentical).[177] However, if your sleep is not getting better at the same time as your other symptoms improve, you may have a sleep disorder such as sleep apnoea or restless leg syndrome. These are quite common in middle-aged women and can be treated once identified.[178]

▶ Depression can significantly affect your ability to sleep, both during and independently of the menopause.[179] Please do seek help from your doctor or a private therapist if you're feeling overwhelmed and consistently under a black cloud.

▶ If you are waking up at night and finding it difficult to get back to sleep, deep breathing exercises may help, particularly diaphragmatic breathing. You'll know if you're breathing through your diaphragm if your tummy extends when breathing in and pulls in when exhaling. Place your hand on your upper chest; it shouldn't move in or out if you're breathing through your diaphragm. Breathe in slowly through your nose for a count of five and repeat the word 'calm'. Exhale slowly to a count of five also. Deep breathing can take practice as shallow chest breathing often develops throughout life. If you find that your chest moves up and down when you breathe and you find diaphragmatic breathing difficult, practise the deep breathing on a daily basis. In addition to helping you sleep, breathing deeply can combat anxiety and promote overall health.

Dealing with relationship difficulties

Challenges can be placed on a relationship during the menopause due to the symptoms, both urogenital and emotional. Mood swings and irritability can lead to trivial arguments which may drive couples apart, even when there are no deep-rooted problems in the relationship. Therefore, if you're feeling that the relationship with your life partner has become strained, consider the advice below.

Educate your partner

The tearfulness, anxiety, and depression that can emerge during the menopause may lead your partner to feel bewildered. Many people (both men and women) don't know a great deal about the myriad of symptoms that can occur during perimenopause, menopause and once you are postmenopausal. And why would they? It's not a topic covered in any great deal in biology lessons at school and anyway, that would have been some time ago. Also, in modern society growing older and the menopause is a somewhat taboo topic and not one that is discussed openly in the media. Therefore, it would be safe to assume that your spouse (particularly male spouses) may know very little about the menopause bar the stereotypical hot flush episodes shown on films. Indeed, there is a serious lack of research on the experiences of partners during this time.

Our suggestion for dealing with this is to share the facts of the menopause with your partner, particularly the range and severity of symptoms that can occur. Humans are meaning-making creatures and so without this information, partners can wonder if they are to blame for changes in mood and diminishing sexual activity. This can lead to a deep sense of confusion and frustration which needn't be the case. By helping your partner understand what you're experiencing, s/he'll be in a better position to support you. Either simply give your spouse this book, or even just the first chapter, to read, or have a frank discussion about what you are experiencing. We appreciate the latter can be difficult so perhaps by letting your partner read some of the material in this book, lines of communication can be opened. There's an enormous amount of material online as well, although bear in mind some of this won't be based on research and evidence.

Sex

As mentioned in Chapter 1, the physiological hormonal changes that women undergo during the menopause can decrease sexual activity. This is not always the case and some women find that the freedom from worrying about possible pregnancies and other aspects of the menopause can be liberating and bring about an enhanced sexual relationship. However, many women do find the urogenital symptoms associated with the menopause, coupled with diminished desire, impact on both the frequency and quality of sex.

Again, communication is key so the first and foremost strategy for tackling sexual difficulties is to discuss them with your partner. Even though HRT (covered in the next two chapters) and the other techniques we covered in previous chapters will help you to manage and often eliminate symptoms, you should not have to deal with any negative consequences of the menopause alone. If you both find it difficult to talk openly, a therapist can help; however we appreciate that visiting a therapist can also be a difficult step to take. But please don't assume that the hormonal dips during the menopause automatically lead to a deteriorating sex life; research has shown that previous sexual function and the feelings of partners are more important than hormonal changes in maintaining sexual function at this stage of life.[180,181]

Stay feeling good – inside and out

In Chapter 1 we also outlined research which demonstrated that rather than physiological variations *per se*, subjective feelings of attractiveness were often related to whether the menopause was perceived as a time of freedom and liberation, or whether it was viewed as a time of relative invisibility. Therefore, using strategies that help to boost positive self-image can be advantageous to maintaining a healthy sex life and also overall good health.

This is of course easier said than done. Nevertheless staying physically active (Chapter 6), accepting the end of fertile years and doing small things that give you a confidence boost (below), will allow you to feel alluring and sexy at any age. Your partner can directly help with this too; this again is something that needs to be tackled in an open, non-judgemental conversation as sometimes comments can be perceived as accusations. For example, rather than saying 'you don't give me compliments like you used to' it is better to express feelings in a less critical manner such as 'I want our relationship to be as good as possible and so it would really help if you told me how sexy you thought I looked'. He or she may be surprised by your directness but will most likely be grateful for it.

A little help from our friends

There is now a wealth of research that shows the importance of social support in health and wellbeing.[181] Social support can come in many forms including practical, emotional, and informational support or even companionship. Theories regarding why social support has a positive impact on health include stress-buffering and psychoneuroimmunology, or PNI, as explained in Chapter 4. PNI research looks at the interaction between psychological, neuroendocrine, and immune systems and has shown that social support is related to optimal functioning in these structures.[182] Considering the increased risk of cardiovascular disease postmenopause, the impact of social support on heart health would seem particularly important to maintaining overall wellbeing at this time of life. The good news is that women are exceptionally good at giving social support so if you're having a difficult time with menopausal symptoms or feeling low in general do reach out to your support network.

Online support groups

Needless to say, many support groups and forums are online these days. If you'd prefer not to discuss your health with your family and friends, online groups can act as a support system. Online support groups offer anonymity, ease of access in terms of place and time, differential perspectives and views, and are often markedly sensitive to embarrassing or stigmatised issues.[183] It's easier to be open and honest when behind a computer screen (known as the disinhibition effect) so if some of your symptoms are challenging to discuss with your partner or friends, online support can be invaluable. Forums and online groups also offer a wealth of informational support but bear in mind not all of this will be evidenced based. Taken together, the benefits of online support groups can generate a sense of empowerment that in turn can lead to improved health.[184]

Take advantage of this time with hobbies and interests

Is there something you've always wanted to do but never felt you had the time or confidence to do it? Perhaps you loved dancing as a child but gave it up when you started work. There are masses of dance classes and most these days don't require a partner, even if they're traditional types (people are simply paired on the day). Or maybe you've thought about doing something creative such as contemporary art but lacked the confidence to try it. Do it now, either via a course or simply by yourself. Seek out and attend lectures and seminars on things that interest you. The internet is awash with forums and groups on every hobby or activity you can imagine. Travel if you're curious about the world, either alone or with a partner. The options are truly limitless here; take advantage of the freedoms that come with this time of life.

Chapter 6 summary and take home messages

In this chapter we've outlined a number of self-help techniques that can be incorporated into your symptom management plan. Most of this advice can be used at any time of life, for any set of symptoms or condition. To recap, the take home messages from this chapter are:

▶ Use a symptom diary to identify patterns and symptom triggers. These can be food, drink, emotional, and situational stressors and can vary day-to-day, month-to-month or over longer periods. Take your completed symptom diary to your doctor or healthcare practitioner as this information will also help them find appropriate treatments for you.

▶ Eating healthily and regularly can aid weight management in addition to exercising and keeping active. Avoid fad and crash diets, low-fat and processed foods, and diet drinks and always eat breakfast. Use your symptom diary to spot comfort eating and try to eat mindfully rather than eating while on the go or working. Finally, pack your diet with fresh fruit and vegetables and allow treats now and then to avoid feeling that food is the enemy.

▶ If you have significant sleep problems even after other menopausal symptoms have improved, discuss this with your doctor to rule out primary sleep disorders. Otherwise, practise sleep hygiene methods and keep the bedroom for sex and sleep only (no devices).

▶ Life transitions can have an impact (both positive and negative) on relationships so, if possible, discuss what you're experiencing with your partner. Do things for yourself to boost confidence and your sense of attractiveness as this can have the secondary consequence of enhancing sexual activity.

▶ Make use of your support networks or online support groups if you prefer. Not only do these offer practical and emotional support, the benefits of social support are far reaching in terms of physical health (particularly cardiovascular health).

▶ Jump into hobbies and interests; if not now, when?

In the next chapter we will explain the history of hormone replacement therapy (HRT), what the difference is between bioidentical and non-bioidentical HRT, the associated benefits and risks, and why HRT has been associated with so much controversy over the years.

Chapter 7

BIOIDENTICAL AND NON-BIOIDENTICAL HORMONE THERAPY

HISTORY AND CONTROVERSIES

Hormone Replacement Therapy (HRT), also called Menopausal Hormone Therapy (MHT), is probably one of the most confusing areas for women and it is not surprising, given the intense media coverage it attracts. Many women have read about the risks which can include a higher likelihood of breast cancer, blood clots, stroke, and heart attack in some women. This can result in a great deal of fear leading to some women not using HRT, whilst others have such debilitating symptoms that they feel they have no choice but to take it, and then worry about the possible side effects. We should stress that not all women need to supplement their hormones. However, if the range of nutritional and lifestyle approaches detailed in Chapters 2–6 do not help to improve your hormone balance and alleviate your symptoms, then HRT is something you may wish to consider. In the next two chapters we will endeavour to give you the facts that you need to make the best decision for your own individual health.

Despite the controversies surrounding the use of HRT, particularly over the last few decades, an estimated one million women in the UK and six million worldwide use some form of HRT to help them manage the symptoms of menopause. The decision on whether to use HRT should be a joint one between you and your doctor, once the benefits and risks have been made clear. Fortunately, this book is timely as new guidelines have just been published by The National Institute for Health and Care Excellence (NICE) in the UK.[185] In addition, in 2013, a Global Consensus Statement on MHT was published, endorsed by a number of prominent medical societies. This included The Endocrine Society, The European Menopause and Andropause Society, The International Menopause Society and The North American Menopause Society,[186] so we are in a position to provide you with the very latest information.

There are no easy answers when it comes to the question of HRT as it will depend on many different factors, including dosage levels and what form the hormone comes in (pill, patch, or cream). Different forms of hormones are recognised differently by our cells and it therefore makes sense that their effects in the body might also be different. We will explain more later about the different preparations available and those used in studies, and why this can make such a difference.

By the end of this chapter, you should be clear about the benefits and risks of HRT. However, it is useful first to have an understanding of what exactly HRT is, how it has changed over the decades, and why it has been so controversial.

What is HRT?

Put simply, HRT replaces the hormones that have rapidly declined as a result of menopause. More recently, it has been called Menopausal Hormone Therapy (MHT) or HT by scientists and researchers. However, we will continue to use the term HRT as this is the one most women are familiar with. As it is used today, HRT is a combination of oestrogen and progestogens, in various formulations. Progestogens (known as progestagens in the USA) is the collective term for both progesterone and synthetic progestins derived from progesterone, or from testosterone. As you will come to understand, progestins have different effects in the body depending on what they are made from (parent molecule). Even very small structural changes in the 'parent molecule' may induce considerable differences in the human body.[187]

What are bioidentical hormones?

The term bioidentical has caused much confusion and controversy, not just amongst the public but within the medical community as well. Some menopause experts prefer the use of the term body-identical as they believe that is more accurate. A group of pharmacists in Canada, after discovering and reviewing over 60 definitions of the term 'bioidentical hormone' in scientific papers and on the internet, proposed the following definition: 'bioidentical hormones are chemical substances that are identical in molecular structure to human hormones'.[188] It is important to realise that 'bioidentical' and 'natural' are not the same thing, even though you will find these terms used interchangeably. For example, the steroids contained in yam or soy cannot be converted within our bodies and have to be converted in a laboratory. They are therefore 'synthetic', which many readers may perceive to be a bad thing. It isn't. The most important factor is that your body recognises the supplemental hormone to be the same molecular structure as that same hormone in your body.

Criticisms

Interest in bioidentical hormones surged, partly as a result of celebrity endorsements (Suzanne Somers, Oprah Winfrey and Gwyneth Paltrow, for example), marketing by compounding pharmacists, and the perception that bioidentical hormones are safer than conventional HRT. We will cover compounding pharmacies and the safety of bioidentical hormones in the next chapter. What we need to emphasise here is that there is nothing wrong with bioidentical hormones if they are sourced correctly and given in the correct dosages, taking into consideration a woman's individual risk profile. However, the protocol (dosing schedule) advocated by Suzanne Somers in her books, called the Wiley Protocol, is controversial and needs further explanation.

What is the Wiley Protocol?

The Wiley Protocol is a scheduled way of taking bioidentical hormones developed by Teresa Wiley (T.S. Wiley), who writes on women's health issues. However, she has no medical qualifications and has been heavily criticised for promoting this protocol without scientific evidence to back it up. The Wiley Protocol gives daily doses of hormones to mimic the peaks and troughs of a 20-year-old, which means a peak of oestrogen at Day 12 which Wiley says 'resets the progesterone receptors' mid-month. This may be the case in younger women, when the high levels of oestrogen in the first half of the cycle are preparing the womb for pregnancy, and then the high levels of progesterone in the second half of the cycle are there to maintain the pregnancy (or levels drop if no ovulation occurs, as explained in Chapter 1, causing the womb lining to shed in preparation for the next cycle). However, we can't bring back ovulation in postmenopausal women and most women past menopause do not want their periods back. The aim of HRT in postmenopausal women is to increase the hormone levels just enough to alleviate symptoms, that is to be on a par with those postmenopausal women who are NOT experiencing symptoms, not restore levels to those of our reproductive years.

Suzanne Somers has written a number of books on the subject of bioidentical hormones, including *Ageless: The Naked Truth about Bioidentical Hormones* (2006), in which she advocates the Wiley Protocol. Following the publication of this book, a number of doctors expressed concerns that women may be harmed by some of the claims made. Although the book is referenced and appears to be backed up by scientific evidence, many of the claims throughout the book are scientifically unproven and therefore potentially harmful to women. The Danish Study that is quoted on the Wiley Protocol website (see Useful Addresses/Websites) as supporting 'the use of cyclically dosed hormone replacement therapy' is misleading. First, this study is not using bioidentical hormones and, second, although it is not made clear in this study exactly how high the levels of oestrogen and progestogen were, they definitely did not use the Wiley Protocol.[189] The Wiley Protocol gives very high levels of oestrogen and progesterone which have not been tested in the long-term and could be dangerous. In fact, there is a website set up by a group of women who believe they have been harmed by this protocol called Rhythmic Living...a cautionary tale about the Wiley Protocol (see Useful Addresses/Websites). So, although women may feel better when first on this protocol, it is really not possible to predict with certainty that this protocol is without side effects and safe long-term. Therefore, we cannot recommend this protocol at this time.

HRT changes and controversy through the decades

HRT has certainly had its fair share of controversy, which we will now summarise to show the major influences, research and how perceptions have changed since 1923, when oestrogenic steroids were first isolated.

1934 Progesterone was discovered.

1944 Russell Marker, a chemist from the University of Pennsylvania, found that diosgenin (from yams) could be converted into progesterone. He then went to Mexico to see if he could find the richest plant source and started setting up companies to produce progesterone in 1944. He refused to sign patent documents because he wanted to make the process of obtaining progesterone from the plant source open to everyone. For a long time, progesterone could only be used in the form of creams or gels because it was rapidly inactivated by the liver if taken orally. However, a form of progesterone known as micronised has been available and widely used in Europe since the 1980s.[190] The term 'micronised' means made into smaller particles (for better absorption).

1941 Premarin, the brand name for the first synthetic oestrogen, was patented and sold as a treatment for menopausal symptoms. Premarin is conjugated oestrogens isolated from the urine of pregnant mares (PREgnant MAre's uRINe).

1966 Robert Wilson's book *Feminine Forever* was published,[191] which sold 100,000 copies in a matter of months. The author stated that women on oestrogen therapy 'will be much more pleasant to live with and will not be dull and unattractive'. Women began to ask their doctors for oestrogen supplementation and Premarin sales escalated.

1969 Psychiatrist Dr David Reuben published his best-selling book called *Everything You Always Wanted to Know About Sex (But Were Afraid to Ask).*[192] Dr Reuben stated that 'as oestrogen is shut off, a [postmenopausal] woman comes as close as she can to being a man' and 'having outlived their ovaries, [postmenopausal women] have outlived their usefulness as human beings'. Once again, Premarin sales escalated.

1969 Professor John Studd started the first menopause clinic in the UK, which was so controversial at the time that the clinic was closed down for three months following protests from the British Medical Association.

1975 The *New England Journal of Medicine* published two studies showing that women who took oestrogen alone without progesterone had four or more times greater risk of endometrial cancer.[193,194] In women with seven or more years of use, there was a 14 times greater risk. In other words, oestrogen alone was dangerous for a woman with a uterus. Doctors began to give Provera (a synthetic progestin) along with oestrogen. In 1980, it was reported in the medical journal *Obstetrics and Gynaecology* that adding progestin to oestrogen led to a decline in endometrial cancer.[195]

1976 A study showed that breast cancer may be increased in oestrogen users. Subsequent studies showed other increased health risks.

1986 The theory that oestrogen protects women from heart disease began to be questioned and studied. The Framingham Heart Study report showed 1234 women taking oestrogen had more cardiovascular events than women who did not use hormones (50 per cent more) and concluded that there was no coronary benefit from oestrogen use. However, the Nurses' Health Study, based on questionnaires sent to 121,964 female nurses aged 30–55, concluded that the risk of heart disease dropped among those who took oestrogen.

1989 A Swedish study of 23,244 women, published in the *New England Journal of Medicine* showed oestrogen replacement therapy caused a slight increase in breast cancer. Further, when women switched to combination HRT (oestrogen and progestin), their breast cancer risk more than doubled.

1990 A large trial called the Postmenopausal Estrogen Progestin Interventions Trial (PEPI) was completed (began 1987), which showed that HRT (non-bioidentical) reduced some risks, such as LDL (the so-called 'bad cholesterol', as explained in Chapter 1) but increased other triglycerides (fats in the blood). The PEPI study was the first major study in the US that compared micronised progesterone (bio-identical) as one of its therapies. Investigators found that micronised progesterone protected the endometrium and did NOT negatively affect fat levels in the blood.

1994 The National Institutes of Health (NIH) authorised a study called the Women's Health Initiative (WHI) involving 25,000 women, followed for eight-and-a-half years, to investigate the long term effects of synthetic HRT (Premarin and Prempro).

1995 The *American Journal of Obstetrics & Gynecology* published an article stating that not only long-term but short-term users of Premarin had a 40 per cent risk of acquiring breast cancer. Although women were concerned, sales kept going strong because of a fear of becoming 'unwomanly'.

1995 The Nurse's Health Study was published. Women taking synthetic oestrogen alone had a 36 per cent increased risk of breast cancer; those on synthetic oestrogen plus progestin had a 50 per cent increase; those on progestins alone had a 240 per cent increased risk.

1998 The HERS Study (Heart and Estrogen-Progestin Replacement Study) showed HRT did not help women who already had a heart attack and may cause more heart attacks and strokes in that group.

Major controversy

2000 The WHI (Women's Health Initiative) was halted to warn women of the preliminary findings. Study participants taking HRT were told that women were experiencing heart attack and strokes and were offered the chance to drop out. The NIH allowed the study to continue, apparently in the hope that the trend would diminish over time.

2002 The WHI study was terminated early due to an increased risk of breast cancer, heart disease, stroke, and blood clots in those women taking the oestrogen/progestin combination. This was accompanied by an enormous amount of media coverage. Doctors were urged to prescribe HRT for short-term relief only.

2004 The oestrogen-only arm of the WHI study was also terminated due to the increased risk of stroke in those women taking conjugated equine (horse-derived) oestrogen. Prescriptions of HRT fell by more than 50 per cent worldwide after these study results were made public.

More than a decade later, researchers and scientists now understand some of the reasons for the negative effects. The WHI study has been heavily criticised as being poorly-designed as it gave HRT to women in their 60s and 70s (average age 63), instead of starting the study when they went through menopause at around 50. Some of the women were also obese, and had heart-related conditions and events, such as heart disease, strokes and high blood pressure. However, since the purpose of the study was to assess health conditions such as heart attack, osteoporosis and stroke, which often do not show up until women are over 60, this would have made the study very long and expensive.

The risks and benefits explained

According to the Global Consensus Statement by the major menopause societies on HRT in 2013, 'the option of HRT is an individual decision in terms of quality of life and health priorities as well as personal risk factors such as age, time since menopause and the risk of venous thromboembolism, stroke, ischemic heart disease and breast cancer'.[196] However, partly due to the way these risks are reported in the media, women have become very confused about exactly what the risks (and benefits) are and how they personally could be affected.

What are the benefits?

Symptom relief

Studies show that nothing beats HRT when it comes to dealing with the symptoms of menopause such as hot flushes and night sweats, associated sleep disturbance, and other issues such as vaginal dryness, pain during intercourse, and frequent urinary tract infections. Furthermore, short-term use of HRT may improve mood and depressive symptoms during perimenopause and in early menopause.[197]

Oestrogen for urinary symptoms and sexual wellbeing

Common menopausal complaints include vaginal dryness, pain during intercourse, and frequent urinary tract infections. These symptoms are often collectively referred to as 'vaginal atrophy' (thinning, drying, and inflammation of the vaginal walls) or 'urogenital atrophy' (changes in the vagina and lower urinary tract) and are due to declining oestrogen levels in these areas. Systemic or topical HRT can improve vaginal lubrication and may help relieve symptoms of urinary frequency and urgency and possibly reduce the risk of recurrent urinary tract infections by up to 60 per cent.[198]

The decision to use systemic or local oestrogen will be influenced by your individual risk of breast cancer or thrombosis and also if in addition you require treatment for vasomotor symptoms, and/or protection from osteoporosis. If urogenital atrophy is the only problem, the most effective treatment is low-dose vaginal oestrogen replacement, in the form of creams, rings, tablets, or pessaries,[199] which can be used long-term as required. Local oestrogen therapy alleviates symptoms such as vaginal dryness and irritation, pain and burning during urination (dysuria), pain (dyspareunia) during sexual activities, urge incontinence and recurrent urinary tract infections.[200, 201] Conjugated equine estrogen (CEE) should not be prescribed, with or without progestin, for the prevention or relief of urinary incontinence (UI) as it has been shown to increase the risk of UI among continent women and worsened UI among symptomatic women after one year.[202] As vaginal oestrogen is low dose and mainly absorbed locally, there is no requirement to combine this with progestogen treatment for endometrial protection. Non-hormonal preparations, such as vaginal moisturisers and lubricants are covered in Chapter 9.

Migraines

Migraines can sometimes be linked to fluctuations in hormones and the menstrual cycle. If you find your migraines are linked to your menstrual cycle (perimenopause), you should see your doctor as they may be able to prescribe a low-dose oestrogen on days surrounding your period as a preventive measure (this may be not be possible if your period is unpredictable, as it often is during perimenopause). Some women on HRT will have a reduction in migraines, while others might have worse symptoms. It is important to work with your doctor to find the right balance.

Osteoporosis

HRT is effective in preserving bone density and preventing osteoporosis in both the spine and hip, as well as reducing the risk of fractures. Studies have estimated between 15 and 25 fewer fragility fractures per 1000 menopausal women, depending on the age of the women studied, the treatment duration and the number of years of follow-up.[203] However, five years after stopping HRT, that risk reverts to what it would have been had you not taken it.

Although HRT is approved for the prevention of osteoporosis in postmenopausal women, it is not currently approved for treatment in postmenopausal women who have no other symptoms.[204] However, it is approved for treatment for women who have had a premature or early menopause, and menopausal women below the age of 60 if they also have menopausal symptoms. After the age of 60, initiating HRT for the sole purpose of the prevention of osteoporotic fractures is not recommended.[205] Therefore, if you are in a high risk group for osteoporosis, you may have to consider other long-term treatments such as bisphosphonates, raloxifene, or strontium ranelate that are generally effective, though not without side effects (see Chapter 9).

Extended use of HRT may be considered acceptable if you have moderate or severe symptoms and are at high risk of osteoporosis. When alternate therapies are not appropriate or have adverse side effects, the extended use of HRT is an option for you if you are at a high risk of osteoporotic fractures.[206]

WHAT DO THE EXPERTS SAY?

All the major menopause societies agree that HRT 'is effective and appropriate for the prevention of osteoporosis-related fractures in at-risk women before age 60 years, or within 10 years after menopause'.[207]

Heart

Before the menopause, women have a much lower risk of heart attack and stroke than men, although this risk becomes the same as men within ten years after the menopause. It was therefore initially assumed that this was related to the drop in oestrogen levels and that restoring premenopausal levels would be protective for the heart. Early studies were promising, suggesting a 50 per cent reduction in risk of Coronary Heart Disease (CHD) in HRT users.[208] The Danish osteoporosis trial showed that HRT reduced the incidence of heart disease by around 50 per cent if started within ten years of the menopause, which is known as the 'window of opportunity' for primary prevention.[209]

However, studies over the years have been conflicting with some showing a neutral impact of HRT on heart risk overall, although certain measures of heart disease risk (those that indicate inflammation and damage) improved.[210] Oestrogen replacement has been found to reduce abdominal obesity, new-onset diabetes, and fat levels in the blood, and improve glucose and insulin metabolism, providing it is prescribed with the right progestogen.[211]

HRT may be protective when given to younger women close to the onset of menopause. A comprehensive review of 19 studies, involving 40,000 women, carried out at the University of Oxford in 2015, reported that starting HRT within ten years of the onset of menopause could cut the risk of early death and heart disease.[212] Most of the early positive studies involved women younger than 55 who had started HRT within two to three years of menopause, whereas in clinical trials, women were aged 63–64. It would appear that women who start HRT within ten years of menopause have a reduced risk of heart disease, whereas those who wait more than ten years have an increased risk.[213]

The 2013 Global Consensus Statement on HRT stated that:

Randomized clinical trials and observational data as well as meta-analyses provide evidence that standard-dose estrogen-alone HRT may decrease coronary heart disease and all-cause mortality in women younger than 60 years of age and within 10 years of menopause. Data on estrogen plus progestogen HRT in this population show a similar trend for mortality but in most randomized clinical trials no significant increase or decrease in coronary heart disease has been found.[214]

Colorectal cancer

Some studies suggest a small reduced risk of colorectal cancer with the use of HRT, although this was only in women taking oral oestrogen (conjugated equine estrogen) combined with a synthetic progestin (MPA). The WHI results found six fewer colorectal cancers per 10000 women per year.[215] There was no reduction in those taking the same oestrogen only.

Diabetes

Although HRT is not licensed or recommended for the prevention of diabetes, a number of trials have shown small reductions in cases of new onset Type 2 diabetes. For example, in the WHI trial, there were 15 fewer cases per 10,000 women per year of therapy (14 fewer in those taking oestrogen only). Other trials have reported similar reductions.[216]

What are the risks?

As well as benefits, HRT has some risks that you will need to consider when you're deciding to take it, or whether to carry on taking it.

An important thing to understand when calculating your own individual risk profile for taking HRT is that 'relative' risk, which is quoted as a percentage and is the most usual way portrayed in the media, always sounds much more alarming than 'actual' risk, which is given as absolute numbers and is the figure you should always pay attention to. For example, a recent media warning of 'a forty per cent increase in risk of ovarian cancer' is an 'actual' risk of 1 in 1000 extra cancer cases and 1 in 1000 extra deaths for those on HRT. However, whilst some women may view 1 in 1000 as a small, or moderate, risk, others may view this as reason not to take HRT, or stop it if they are already taking it. Another important consideration is that our risks of contracting certain health conditions increases with age (baseline risk), so it is always important to separate the potential increased risk should you choose to take HRT.

When it comes to evaluating your own individual risk profile of taking HRT, the following will also need to be taken into account:

▶ how severe your symptoms are

▶ how your quality of life is affected

▶ personal and family health history

▶ your own attitude to risk and your priorities in life. For example, some people would rather take calculated risks and have a full and happy life than live a risk-free life but have their symptoms affect their lifestyle.

Hence, taking HRT is an individual choice and the pros and cons may be very different from one woman to another. This is one reason why we advise that you speak in detail with your doctor or specialist about these risks and the benefits that apply to you personally. You may want to try using the other strategies we discuss in previous chapters first, before embarking on HRT treatment.

Breast cancer

The risk of breast cancer associated with HRT has been widely reported in the media and is still very much an area of controversy. Combined HRT use beyond three to five years is associated with an increased risk of breast cancer, whereas recent evidence shows that oestrogen alone has little impact, unless used for longer than 15 years. This is surprising, given early studies. Also, only women who have had their uterus removed can take oestrogen alone.

For decades, researchers were aware that both oestrogen and progesterone had the potential to stimulate growth of breast cells. By the early 1990s, it was well known that oestrogens promoted the growth of breast cancer.[217] In the late 1980s and early 1990s, there was great concern over the long-term influence of oral contraceptives on the development of breast cancer in women.[218] Oestrogens were known to stimulate the growth of breast cancer cells and so too were certain progestins, but not all. A number of laboratory and animal studies were carried out to investigate this but study results were conflicting.

Human studies have also been conflicting. Some report on risk based on duration of use, some based on age, others based on the different types and dosages of HRT used. When study results are reported in the media, it is rarely made clear exactly what type of HRT and dosages were used, and why this could make a difference. For example, some study results, particularly in the last ten years, suggest that the risk of breast cancer is higher if oestrogen is combined with synthetic progestins (such as medroxyprogesterone acetate (MPA), which is the progestin used in many studies), rather than micronised progesterone (bioidentical).

RISK BASED ON DURATION OF USE

In 1997, a group of researchers reanalysed about 90 per cent of the worldwide evidence on the link between HRT and breast cancer risk.[219] They calculated that in North America and Europe, the number of cases of breast cancer in women between the ages of 50 and 70 who had *never used HRT* is about 45 per 1000 women. The estimated additional cases of breast cancer for women who started HRT at age 50 were:

▶ two extra cases per 1000 women (five years of use)

▶ six extra cases per 1000 women (ten years of use)

▶ 12 extra cases per 1000 women (15 years of use).

What was interesting to note, however, was that although the risk of having breast cancer diagnosed increased for each year of HRT use, the risk of breast cancer increased by a similar factor for each year older at menopause amongst women who had never used HRT. Whether HRT affects mortality from breast cancer was not known from this study.

The Million Women Study (MWS) was a questionnaire survey by Cancer Research UK of women attending the National Health Service breast screening programme.[220] This was reported by the media as a 'doubling of risk of breast cancer' with HRT, failing to mention the absolute risk of:

▶ one-and-a-half extra cases of breast cancer per 1000 women after five years of use (oestrogen-only therapy)

▶ six extra cases of breast cancer per 1000 women after five years of use (oestrogen/progestogen therapy).

These extra cases are in addition to the baseline risk of 32 cases in 1000 women aged 50–64.

Estimates from the 2015 NICE Guideline, when looking at the difference in breast cancer incidence per 1000 postmenopausal women over a period of seven-and-a-half years (baseline risk 22.48 per 1000), revealed:

▸ four more cases for less than five years treatment; five more cases for five to ten years treatment (oestrogen alone)

▸ 12 more cases for less than five years treatment; 21 more cases for five to ten years treatment (oestrogen + progestogen).

It should be noted, however, that these figures are based on grouping together a number of observational studies, covering a wide age range, and also a wide range of different preparations.[221]

RISK BASED ON AGE

The Women's Health Initiative (WHI) is one of the most quoted studies when it comes to investigating the link between breast cancer and HRT use. As previously noted, this study was stopped prematurely due to an excess number of breast cancer cases.[222] Some have attributed the fall in breast cancer rates in the USA since 2002 to the drop-off in HRT use following the results of this study. However, this has since been criticised by menopause societies, saying that rates were starting to fall anyway prior to 2002 and this may have occurred because the women who stopped taking HRT were no longer attending breast screening. The results from the WHI study suggested:[223]

▸ six extra cases of breast cancer per 10,000 women aged 50–59

▸ eight extra cases of breast cancer per 10,000 women aged 60–69

▸ 15 extra cases of breast cancer per 10,000 women aged 70–79.

It is already difficult to compare these figures with the 1997 analysis, which calculates the risk based on the number of years HRT was taken, rather than breaking it down into specific age groups. Also, the results of this study have since been criticised by many prominent researchers due to the factors below:

▶ The average age of women in the study was 63.

▶ Some had already taken HRT before (incidence was not increased in women who had never used any HRT before entering the trial).[224]

▶ Some were taking HRT for the first time up to ten years since menopause, whereas the majority of women seeking help for menopausal symptoms do so either very close to the onset of menopause or during the perimenopausal stage.

▶ The WHI was meant to be a study of 'healthy' women, whereas 30 per cent had a BMI of 30 or above, and 70 per cent had a pre-existing heart disease.[225]

▶ There have been several re-evaluations of the findings from the WHI, causing some to conclude that 'over-interpretation and misrepresentation of the WHI findings have damaged the health and well-being of menopausal women by convincing them and their health professionals that the risks of HRT outweigh the benefits'.[226]

▶ A Danish study, involving 78,380 women aged 40–67, found that HRT did not increase the risk of breast cancer in women aged 40–49, although they did find an increased risk in the over 50s – that increased with duration of use and decreased with time since last prescription.[227]

RISK ASSOCIATED WITH DIFFERENT TYPES OF HRT

The findings of the WHI study, in women using oestrogen alone (those with prior hysterectomy), suggest a possible reduction in breast cancer, which the authors say warrants further investigation.[228] The type of HRT and the dosages used in the WHI study (continuous combined conjugated equine oestrogens (CEE) 0.625mg and medroxyprogesterone acetate (MPA) 2.5mg) have since been called in to question by some researchers, as other formulations/combinations may be safer. Recent trials indicate that bioidentical progesterone combined with oestrogen 'confers less or even no risk of breast cancer as opposed to the use of other synthetic progestins'.[229]

In 2008, a large French study following over 80,000 women for over eight postmenopausal years was published, which concluded that it could be preferable to use bioidentical progesterone or dydrogesterone in order to diminish or eliminate the increased risk of breast cancer. If a woman used micronised progesterone (bioidentical) in combination with oestrogen, there was no increase in risk of breast cancer. There was a slight increased risk if oestrogen was combined with dydrogesterone, which is a synthetic progestin with the closest chemical structure and effects to progesterone. The risk increased in those taking oestrogen alone, with the highest risk being when oestrogen was combined with other progestogens.

In a Danish study, where all female nurses aged 45 and above received questionnaires between 1993 and 1999, the risk was almost double when oestrogen was used alone, but highest when oestrogen was combined with testosterone-like progestins. This study provides further evidence that the type of progestin and dosing regimen used does make a difference.[230]

Many researchers have suggested that micronised progesterone may be the optimal choice as part of combined HRT[231] and that it does not increase cell growth in breast tissue in postmenopausal women compared with MPA, as used in the WHI study.[232] This has been supported in animal studies.[233]

WHAT DO THE EXPERTS SAY?

The consensus of the major menopause societies globally is:

> The risk of breast cancer in women over 50 years associated with HRT is a complex issue. The increased risk of breast cancer is primarily associated with the addition of a progestogen to estrogen therapy and related to the duration of use. The risk of breast cancer attributable to HRT is small and the risk decreases after treatment is stopped.[234]

Take home message regarding breast cancer risk

▶ Women who have breast cancer, or have had breast cancer in the past, should not take HRT.

▶ Taking HRT for five years or more slightly increases the risk of breast cancer. However, the risk for a postmenopausal women taking HRT for five years is about the same as for a woman of the same age who is still having periods over that time and not taking HRT (later menopause).

▶ Long-term use of HRT is associated with an increased risk of breast cancer and the risk goes up the longer you take it. However, if you stop HRT, after about five years your risk has largely, if not wholly, disappeared and becomes the same as a woman of the same age who never took HRT.

▶ The risk for a woman taking oestrogen plus progestogen HRT is higher than for oestrogen-only HRT. However, only women who no longer have a womb can use oestrogen-only HRT, as progestogens protect the womb lining. There is increasing evidence to suggest that micronised progesterone (bioidentical) is not associated with an increased risk of breast cancer. Although evidence is not yet conclusive that bioidentical hormones are completely safe and it is important to be aware of this, it makes sense, in our opinion, to avoid synthetic progestins and ask your doctor for bioidentical progesterone (micronised).

Whether you decide to take HRT or not, it is always important to examine your breasts regularly, as advised in Chapter 1, and consider breast screening if you are at risk or over 50.

Heart and circulation

It was initially thought that oestrogen would be protective for the heart. This may still be the case if HRT is prescribed at the lowest possible dose as close to the onset of menopause as possible (and therefore under the age of 60), known as 'the window of opportunity'.[235, 236] However, it is now believed that oestrogen loses its protective effect if initiated far from the onset on menopause, especially if there is unstable plaque in the arteries.[237]

Increased risk of blood clots and stroke

When studies are carried out to investigate possible associations between HRT and heart disease, some studies look at blood clots, others at stroke.

BLOOD CLOTS

HRT may increase the risk of blood clots in the veins (also called deep vein thrombosis or DVT), especially during the first year of taking it. These blood clots are not always serious, but if one travels to the lungs, it can cause chest pain, breathlessness, collapse, or even death. This is called pulmonary embolism, or PE. Both DVT and PE are examples of a condition called venous thromboembolism, or VTE. The risk of VTE increases with age, especially in women over 60 and occurs in approximately one per 100 person years in postmenopausal women. It accounts for about one third of all potentially fatal cardiovascular events in postmenopausal women using HRT. Oral contraceptives and Selective Estrogen Recepter Modulators (SERMs) (see Chapter 9) also carry this increased risk, particularly during the first two years of use.[238]

In the University of Oxford review of 40 studies mentioned above, when they looked at women under 60, or those beginning HRT less than a decade after the menopause, they found a reduction in deaths and heart disease but an increase in blood clots and a possible increase in strokes, which suggests that overall the therapy does not protect the heart. Those who started HRT less than 10 years after menopause had lower mortality and heart disease though were still at an increased risk of blood clots (VTE) compared to placebo or no treatment.[239] Henry Boardman, of the department of cardiovascular medicine, who led the review, said that this supported the theory that starting HRT earlier could delay blocking of the arteries, but starting it once arterial furring had set in increased the risk of dangerous blood clots. Dr Boardman said:

> When we looked at the results according to the age of women, or by how long since their menopause that they started treatment, we found that if 1000 women under 60 years old started hormone therapy we would expect six fewer deaths, eight fewer cases of heart disease, and five

extra blood clots over about seven years, compared to 1000 similar women who did not start hormone therapy.

Although it is now well established that oral oestrogen increases the risk of VTE, with the highest risk in the first year of use,[240] a low dose of transdermal oestrogen with or without progesterone / a progestogen does not seem to be associated with the same risk. There is increasing evidence that risk is greater in combination with certain progestogens, such as nomegestrol acetate or promegestone. In comparison, dydrogesterone, medroxyprogesterone acetate, and progesterone were not associated with an increased risk and appear to be safe.[245] The latest advice is that the most suitable options, particularly for high risk individuals (for example, if you have a personal or family history of VTE, or are obese) include micronised progesterone or dydrogesterone.[242]

How likely is a blood clot?

Although blood clots usually happen within one to two years of starting HRT, the magnitude of risk seems to decrease with time. As with other risks, the risk was found to be lower in women who started HRT before the age of 60.

▸ If you look at women in their 50s for an average of five years, in those not taking HRT the risk of a blood clot is about three in 1000. In women taking HRT, seven in 1000 would be expected to get a blood clot. So, four extra cases.

▸ If you look at women in their 60s for an average of five years, in those not taking HRT, the risk of a blood clot is about eight in 1000. In women taking HRT, 17 in 1000 would be expected to get a blood clot. So, nine extra cases.

You are more likely to get a blood clot if you are seriously overweight; you have had a blood clot before; if a close family member has had blood clots; or if you are off your feet for a long time because of major surgery, injury, or illness. If you get painful swelling in your leg, sudden chest pain, or difficulty breathing, see a doctor as soon as possible.

STROKE

Studies linking HRT and stroke have been conflicting. The WHI study results overall showed an increase in stroke incidence in those using HRT, with eight additional strokes per 10,000 women per year in the oestrogen-only group; and 11 additional strokes per 10,000 women per year in those taking oestrogen with progestin.[243] However, re-analysis of the data has revealed that there was a smaller incidence in women between the ages of 50 and 59, and the increase in risk for stroke was clearly age-related: [244]

▶ four extra cases per 10,000 women per year aged 50–59

▶ nine extra cases per 10,000 women per year aged 60–69

▶ 13 extra cases per 10,000 women per year aged 70–79.

If you are over 60 and have a risk factor for stroke or blood clots, HRT may not be suitable for you.[245] As discussed previously, current evidence suggests that the transdermal route may be better than taking it orally when it comes to stroke risk.

Coronary Heart Disease (CHD)

When the results from the WHI study were first published, it was concluded that overall health risks exceeded benefits from use of combined oestrogen plus progestin for an average follow-up of 5.2 years. The excess risk for women taking combined oestrogen plus progestin was calculated to be seven more CHD events per 10,000 women per year.[246] However, there was no increase in heart disease in the group of women with prior hysterectomy, and therefore taking oestrogen-only. In April 2007, data from the WHI study were reanalysed and published, showing that there was no increase in heart disease in the younger group, aged 50–59 years.[247]

All the major menopause societies globally agree that the risk of VTE and stroke increases with oral HRT but the absolute risk is rare below age 60 years. Studies point to a lower risk with transdermal therapy.[248]

Gallbladder disease

Gallbladder disease, which includes gallstones (cholelithiasis) and inflammation of the gallbladder (cholecystitis), is common in middle aged women and the use of HRT increases the risk. However, results of the Million Women Study (MWS), published in the British Medical Journal in 2008, reported a substantially lower risk of gallbladder disease with the use of transdermal, rather than oral, oestrogen HRT.[249]

In the UK over five years an estimated 1.1 per cent of middle-aged women who have never used HRT are admitted to hospital for a cholecystectomy (removal of the gallbladder). Use of transdermal oestrogen increases the risk to 1.3 per cent and use of oral oestrogens increases this to 2 per cent. Among users of oral HRT, the risk increased with higher doses compared to lower doses, and the use of equine oestrogen was associated with a slightly higher risk than oestradiol. The risk has been found to decrease with time since stopping HRT. Transdermal oestrogens are generally prescribed in lower doses than oral and are absorbed through the skin and directly into the circulation. The MWS researchers concluded that for women who choose to use HRT, the use of transdermal therapy rather than oral therapy over a five-year period could avoid one cholecystectomy in every 140 users.[250]

Ovarian cancer

Ovarian cancer is the fourth most common cancer in women in the UK, with about 6700 cases and 4600 dying from it every year. However, published data on the role of HRT and risk of ovarian cancer are conflicting. Although the risk seems to consistently increase after ten years of HRT use, some studies show no elevated risk with less than ten years of oestrogen therapy, whereas others show there is a risk with less than five years of use.[251] Several studies show a significant increase in risk with oestrogen-only HRT, and a smaller or no increased risk with combined oestrogen and progestogen.[252]

Results from the UK Million Women Study showed that current users of HRT were more likely to develop and die from ovarian cancer than women who had never used it. This incidence increased with increasing duration of use, but did not differ by type of preparation used, its constituents, or mode of administration. As with other risks, the risk of ovarian cancer has been found to decrease with time since stopping HRT and the MWS showed that past users of HRT were not at an increased risk of ovarian cancer. Over five years, the incidence rates equated to one extra ovarian cancer in roughly 2500 users, and one extra ovarian cancer death in roughly 3300 users.[253]

In February 2015, research by the University of Oxford, published in the Lancet (and widely reported by the media), found there was an extra case of ovarian cancer for every 1000 women who had taken HRT for five years from age 50.[254] Professor Richard Peto advises that women should make sure they are aware of the symptoms (bloating, abdominal pain, feeling full, and needing to go to the toilet more often) and speak to their GP if they are concerned. He says short-term (two to five years) use is preferable to longer-term use of HRT.

HRT may not be right for you if you have a family history of ovarian cancer, or have an associated gene mutation such as BRCA.

Endometrial cancer

There is no doubt that oestrogen therapy alone increases the risk of endometrial cancer. This risk is largely avoided by the addition of a progestogen for all or part of the month (depending on whether you are pre- or postmenopausal), although long-term use, for more than five years, may be associated with a small increase in risk.[255] The MWS showed a risk of 3 cases per 1000 women after five years.[256]

Lung cancer

Some studies have associated HRT use with increased lung cancer risk, while others have shown no effect or found lower lung cancer risk in HRT users. Results from the WHI showed that lung cancer rates did not increase in the HRT group, although the number of deaths from lung cancer did increase among treated women (73 vs 40 deaths in the placebo group).[257] However, women taking HRT for short periods for severe menopausal symptoms should remember that the absolute lung cancer risk from HRT remains small (less than 1 per cent), unless you have risk factors, such as being a current or ex-smoker.

Alzheimer's disease/dementia

Studies investigating the link between HRT and dementia show mixed results. Some show improvement in cognitive function with HRT started in early menopause and a possible reduction in the long-term risk of Alzheimer's and dementia.[258] One study found that HRT initiated prior to the final menstrual period had a beneficial effect whereas initiation after the final menstrual period had a detrimental effect on cognitive performance.[259] A review in 2012 grouped together the results of 23 studies, which showed an increased risk of dementia among women over the age of 65, after four years of use.[260] Results from the WHI reported a 'two-fold increase in risk of all-cause dementia' although the average age in this study was 63 and 21 per cent were over 70.[261] It is not recommended that women take HRT as a way to reduce their risk of developing dementia.

Does HRT reduce life expectancy?

In 2004, a group of researchers pooled data from 30 trials from 1966 to 2002 (26,708 women) to determine if there were more, or fewer, deaths from heart disease, cancer, or other causes in those using HRT. They found that HRT reduced the total number of deaths in the younger age group (when average age was under 60), but not in the group over 60 years of age. For all ages combined though, HRT did not affect the risk for death from heart disease or cancer, but reduced deaths from other causes.[262] Results from the WHI study reported two additional deaths per 10,000 women per year attributed to breast cancer, and two additional deaths per 10,000 women per year attributed to all causes, in those taking oestrogen with progestogen who were followed up for 11 years.[263]

WHAT DO THE EXPERTS SAY?

'The use of transdermal oestradiol and micronized progesterone could reduce or possibly even negate the excess risk of VTE, stroke, cholecystitis, and possibly even breast cancer associated with oral use of HRT'[264] and 'in specific clinical settings the choice of the transdermal route of administration of oestrogens and the use of natural progesterone might offer significant benefits and added safety'.[265] Guidelines from the major menopause societies around the globe all contain positive statements regarding transdermal oestradiol and micronised progesterone. Unlike oral oestrogens, transdermal oestradiol has been shown not to increase the risk of VTE, or stroke at doses of 50mcg or less, and to confer a significantly lower risk for gallbladder disease.

Chapter 7 summary

All the major menopause societies agree that 'HRT is the most effective treatment for vasomotor symptoms associated with menopause at any age, but benefits are more likely to outweigh risks for symptomatic women before the age of 60 years or within 10 years after menopause'.[266]

In the next chapter, we will give you information on different types and dosages of HRT in order to help you decide if HRT is right for you.

Chapter 8

WHAT TYPE OF HRT IS RIGHT FOR ME?

Now that you have the information about the risks and benefits of HRT, this chapter will explain the different forms of treatment that you may want to consider. As throughout this book, we strongly recommend that you discuss these options with your doctor or specialist, especially if you are taking any nutrients, such as herbs or phytoestrogen supplements, which also have an effect on your hormone balance. We would also stress that although some hormones (such as progesterone creams) are available via the internet, we strongly advise you against this as it is very important to get the correct dosage and balance. HRT can be used in conjunction with the other types of treatments and therapies that we've outlined in this book and in addition to the general lifestyle practices as set out in Chapter 2. Using the self-help techniques in Chapter 6 will also benefit not only menopausal symptoms, but overall health. There are numerous options when it comes to HRT which we now explain in detail.

When should I start HRT?

Current medical guidelines state that HRT should be prescribed at the lowest dose for the shortest time possible and started as close to menopause as possible. The decision will take into account the severity of your symptoms and the effect on your quality of life, your personal and family history, and your own attitude to risk.

How long should I take it for?

A standard course of HRT for menopausal symptoms is anywhere from two to five years, although it can be continued for as long as the benefits outweigh the risks. The recommendation for duration of therapy for oestrogen combined with a progestogen is limited by the increased risk of breast cancer and breast cancer mortality associated with three to five years of use. However, there is more flexibility in duration of use for oestrogen alone (which is only recommended for women without a uterus), which has a more favourable benefit–risk profile, as observed during an average of seven years of use and four years of follow-up.[267]

What about stopping it?

If HRT is stopped abruptly, symptoms such as hot flushes are likely to return with a vengeance so it is advisable to reduce the dose slowly over several months. This should be discussed with your doctor but is usually over a period of three months or so.

How do I take it?

There are many different doses and different methods of taking HRT, depending on your risk profile and your own individual preference. These include:

▶ transdermal, which are absorbed through the skin and include creams, gels, and patches

▶ vaginal creams, rings, and intravaginal gels

▶ oral, which include tablets, capsules, and drops (that can be taken under the tongue for example)

▶ subcutaneous (implants).

The difference between oral and transdermal is that oral preparations have to first pass through the digestive tract and the liver before entering into the bloodstream, whereas transdermal HRT passes directly into the bloodstream. Ultimately, you and your doctor need to decide what is right for you.

What hormones are used in HRT?

Oestrogen

Oestrogen comes in three main forms:

▶ *Oestradiol (E2)*, or 17 beta (β)-oestradiol, is the form used in most HRT.

▶ *Oestrone (E1)* is the predominant form of oestrogen in your postmenopausal years, if you're not taking HRT, and is not included as part of conventional HRT.

▶ *Oestriol (E3)* is the weakest form of oestrogen, and has been reported to have a protective effect against breast cancer. It is not part of conventional HRT and can only be prescribed by a doctor specialising in bioidentical hormones who uses a compounding pharmacy (see page 189).

Possible side effects of oestrogen

Like all medicines, oestrogen can cause side effects, although not everybody will experience them. Side effects that are considered to be common include:

▶ itching of the vagina or genital area

▶ periods beginning again, including changing menstrual bleeding pattern for up to six months, spotting, prolonged or heavier vaginal bleeding, or vaginal bleeding completely stopping by ten months

▶ pain during intercourse

▶ vaginal discharge.

Any side effect that has ever been reported must be recorded, even if they have only occurred in a small percentage of people. Rather than list them all here, we would just stress that nobody knows your body better than you, so if you are at all concerned, you should contact your doctor. Some may need medical attention and should be reported immediately, such as chest pain, palpitations, high blood pressure, and urinary problems, such as difficulty urinating or urinary tract infection, You should also report any changes in the breasts, such as redness, swelling, tenderness or pain, discharge from the nipple, dimpling of the breast skin, inverted nipple, or lump in the breast or under the arm.

Progestogens

When oestrogen was first used to treat the symptoms of the menopause, it was used alone. However, it was later discovered that oestrogen taken alone increased the risk of cancer of the womb lining and that progesterone, or progestins (known collectively as progestogens), protected the womb lining. Therefore, unless you have had a hysterectomy and no longer have a womb, oestrogen must be combined with a progestogen, to keep the womb lining thinner and to stop it building up to a possibly pre-cancerous level.

The two main types of progestogen currently used in HRT are:

▶ those most closely resembling progesterone (dydrogesterone, drospirenone medroxyprogesterone acetate, and micronized progesterone)

▶ those derived from testosterone (norethisterone, norgestrel, and levonorgestrel).

Possible side effects of progestogens

▶ fluid retention

▶ acne and hirsutism (excessive hair growth such as beard or chest hair – more an issue with testosterone-derived progestins)

▶ mood swings and PMS-like effects.

If side effects are experienced on one type, changing the type or route of progestogen may help. These side effects can be reduced by using micronised progesterone (not suitable for those with a soya allergy because it contains soya lecithin). Using progestogens vaginally (for example progesterone gel and pessaries), provides adequate protection for the womb lining with reduced side effects.[268]

Other reported side effects are similar to those with oestrogen. Many may only occur in a small percentage of people and may diminish once the body becomes used to the medication. Some may need medical attention and should be reported immediately, as detailed above.

How do I take progestogens?

The duration, frequency, and type of progestogen will be determined by your age, and whether you are still having periods (perimenopausal), or if you are postmenopausal (at least one year after your last period). If you have had an early or premature menopause (POI), hormone therapy should generally continue at least until the estimated age of natural menopause (on average 51 years).

Taking progestogen during the perimenopause

If you are still having periods and your last period was less than one year ago, you will be prescribed what is called a 'sequential combined regimen', which means that you will take continuous oestrogen, with progestogen for 12–14 days per month. This will induce a monthly bleed in most women.

Taking progestogen during postmenopause

If you are postmenopausal (i.e. your last period was more than a year ago), you will be prescribed what is called a 'continuous combined regimen', which means you take both oestrogen and a progestogen continually throughout the month. The aim of this regimen is *not* to induce monthly bleeding and to also minimise the risk of endometrial cancer. Your doctor will decide which is best for you. You should always report any bleeding to your doctor so that they can either adjust your dosage or, if necessary, investigate the cause.

Taking progestogen during premature or early menopause

If you have been diagnosed with POI, or experienced menopause early, HRT simply replaces ovarian hormones that should normally be produced at this age and the aim is to replace hormones as close to physiological levels as possible. Therefore, HRT is usually advised until the average age of menopause when treatment should be reassessed.[269] Women experiencing premature menopause are at increased risk of osteoporosis and, possibly, heart disease and dementia, and they often experience more intense symptoms than women reaching menopause naturally. HRT is strongly recommended to control vasomotor symptoms, minimise risk of heart disease, osteoporosis, and possibly Alzheimer's disease, as well as to maintain sexual function. Although the contraceptive pill can be used as an alternative to control symptoms, it is not known if this will be adequate to protect against osteoporosis and heart disease.[270]

Taking progestogen via an Intrauterine system (IUS)
Intrauterine systems, or IUSs, are small, T-shaped devices made of flexible plastic that are inserted by a specially trained doctor or nurse into a woman's womb. Not only is it a contraceptive, but it also releases a small amount of progestogen hormone to the womb lining, making it thinner and hence making heavy periods lighter. In addition to being one of your options to protect your womb lining whilst on oestrogen therapy, hormonal IUSs may reduce period pain and cramps (dysmenorrhoea) and make your period lighter. On average, menstrual flow is reduced by 90 per cent.[271] For some women, periods stop altogether.

THE MIRENA COIL

One particular type of IUS, called the Levonorgestrel releasing-intrauterine system (or Mirena coil), is licensed for heavy bleeding (menorrhagia) and to provide endometrial protection for perimenopausal and postmenopausal women on oestrogen replacement therapy. This is because it releases 20mcg of a progestin (levonorgestrel) per day directly into the uterine cavity.

The Mirena is effective for birth control for five years. IUSs work mainly by affecting the way sperm move so they can't join with an egg, and therefore pregnancy cannot happen. Progestin also prevents pregnancy by thickening a woman's cervical mucus, which blocks sperm and keeps it from joining with an egg.

The Mirena is particularly helpful when periods are heavy (your periods may initially become heavier, longer, or more painful, although this usually improves after a few months); when contraception is still required along with HRT; and when there are side effects from the progestogen part of HRT. However, it may not be suitable for all women. Some women may find it invasive; some experience mild to moderate pain when the IUS is put in, and cramping or backache for a few days after insertion; there may be spotting between periods, and/or irregular periods, in the first three to six months, although this usually settles.

Testosterone

Testosterone has been shown to result in significant improvement in sexual function, including sexual desire and orgasm[272] and can be prescribed if low sexual desire and/or tiredness are an issue for you.

Low sexual desire is a common menopausal problem, although many women are reluctant to discuss it, particularly with their doctor. It is important to realise that this is a common problem, affecting not just women in the menopausal years. It can be an extremely distressing condition and have a range of negative effects on a woman's health and wellbeing. When associated with distress and/or relationship difficulties, it is termed hypoactive sexual desire disorder (HSDD), which is estimated to affect approximately one in ten women, of all ages. Several studies show that the prevalence of HSDD is greater in surgically menopausal women, compared with premenopausal and naturally menopausal women. Women who have had both their ovaries removed can experience a decrease of circulating testosterone levels by 40–50 per cent. Other underlying causes, besides age and menopausal status, can include stress, relationship difficulties, insomnia, fatigue, issues with body image, and side effects of certain medications, such as antidepressants, antipsychotics, and antihypertensives. Please explore these other underlying causes with your doctor if HSDD is an issue for you as there are many options for treatment depending on the cause, for instance psychological therapies or changing medications that result in HSDD.

Possible side effects of testosterone

Side effects, such as acne and excessive hair growth, can be minimised as long as testosterone levels are maintained within the female physiological range. Although at present testosterone is not licensed for female use, testosterone gels licensed for male use are available and your doctor should be able to prescribe lower doses for you. Another option is to see a doctor who specialises in this area and they will be able to prescribe either a testosterone gel (such as Testogel or Testim) or cream via a specialist compounding pharmacy. Many specialists advise low dosages and/or use on alternate days.

Dehydroepiandrosterone (DHEA)

DHEA is often described as part of HRT, as it is a steroid hormone produced by the adrenal gland and converted in the body into various different hormones including oestrogen and testosterone. In the USA, it is classed as a food supplement and available without a prescription, where it is often bought over-the-counter. Levels of DHEA decline with age and using a supplement can be useful in patients who have low levels. Sometimes DHEA may be prescribed if testosterone levels are low but it is really at the judgement of your doctor, depending on test results and how low testosterone is.

Some studies have shown benefits for the bones, brain health, and general wellbeing. However, a review of DHEA studies reported inconsistent results, small sample sizes, and short treatment duration and more recent trials do not support a benefit of oral DHEA therapy for women.[273] However, there is some evidence that vaginal DHEA may help libido through improvement of vaginal dryness, and benefits in relation to desire, arousal, orgasm, and pain were found when used daily for 12 weeks.[274]

DHEA is not available in the UK, although it is possible to have DHEA prescribed at your doctor's discretion ('off licence'). This should be discussed with your doctor if this is something you are considering.

What is HRT made from?

This will depend on whether the hormones are bioidentical or non-bioidentical, as explained in the last chapter.

Oestrogen

When artificial oestrogens were originally made available in the 1920s, they were isolated from the urine of pregnant women, and later from the urine of pregnant mares (you will often see these written as conjugated equine estrogens, or CEE). Later forms have been isolated from plant sources (soy and yams), although the equine type is still widely used and prescribed today, despite criticisms. It is known that CEE contains some oestrogens that are specific to horses and therefore foreign to humans (equilins for example) and there are still many uncertainties about the exact components of the urine extract and what it metabolises into in the human body. Equilin metabolites, for example, appear to have stronger carcinogenic effects than those from oestradiol, which is a concern as they can be involved in the development of hormone-dependent tumours, such as breast cancer. The equine oestrogens equilin and equilenin, both components of Premarin, are metabolised to a chemical (4-hydroxyequilenin) which has been found to cause DNA damage in rats and therefore has the potential to cause cancer.[275] Some experts argue that, since oestradiol is now available in pure form, it seems more sensible to replace the oestradiol deficiency by giving the exact hormone rather than an extract of uncertain composition and that the use of CEE should now be considered inappropriate.[276]

Progesterone

Progesterone is made in the laboratory from either soybeans or the Mexican wild yam. The process was discovered in the 1930s by Professor Russell Marker, of Pennsylvania State University, who transformed diosgenin, steroids contained in wild yams (Dioscorea villosa), to progesterone (the natural form found in humans).

Yam scam

A word of caution: not all products containing 'wild yam extract' actually contain any progesterone. The human body cannot convert the steroids contained in yam to progesterone. This has to be done in a laboratory. It is therefore advisable that you avoid creams derived from wild yam (often widely available online) that are marketed as 'progesterone' creams. Even if they *do* contain any progesterone, it is often impossible to tell how much and how well it will be absorbed.

Bioidentical hormone options (BHRT)

Approved and licensed BHRT

It is important to realise that there are some bioidentical hormones which are licensed and approved by the appropriate regulatory authority in any given country. In the US, this is the FDA; in the UK, the Medicines & Healthcare Products Regulatory Agency (MHRA); and in Europe, the European Medicines Agency (EMA). When the FDA and other regulatory authorities warn against them, they are actually referring to hormones that are prepared at compounding pharmacies. Although the British Menopause Society (BMS) does not recommend compounded hormones due to lack of evidence for efficacy and safety, it does support the use of regulated bioidentical oestradiol, progesterone, and testosterone, which 'may have some advantages over non-identical varieties of HRT'.[277] To help you, we have set out below the main bioidentical hormones available which have been licenced to date:

OESTROGEN

17 beta-oestradiol (from plants and micronised) is a bioidentical oestrogen. In the 1990s, pharmaceutical companies started developing and patenting methods of administering bioidentical hormones. One example is the Climara patch (patented 1994), which uses a sticky transdermal hormone delivery system. Since the oestrogen is identical to human oestradiol, and cannot be patented, the patent was obtained by patenting the glue.

17 beta-oestradiol is available as a patch, a pill, transdermal gel or topical cream, vaginal creams, tablets and rings. Please note that there are some preparations that combine bioidentical oestradiol with non-bioidentical progesterone (a progestin) so, if you are looking for completely bioidentical, these should be avoided. Table 8.1 shows examples of UK and US brand names for the different routes of administration.

TABLE 8.1 EXAMPLES OF UK AND US BRAND NAMES FOR BHRT

	UK	US
17 beta-oestradiol		
Patch	Evorel, Estraderm	Alora, Climara, Esclim, Estraderm, Vivelle
Pill	Estrace	Estrace
Transdermal gel/ cream	Oestrogel	Estradiol, EstroGel, Estrasorb
Vaginal cream, tablet or ring	Estrace	Estrace
Micronized Progesterone		
Pill	Utrogestan	Prometrium
Vaginal pessaries/gel	Utrogestan	Prochieve

PROGESTERONE

One of the most effective forms of bioidentical progesterone is micronised progesterone, which comes in pill form, and as vaginal pessaries/gel, as shown in Table 8.1. Micronised progesterone has been used widely in Europe since 1980 and is well tolerated with the main side effect being mild and transient drowsiness, an effect minimised by taking it at bedtime. Some experts recommend oral micronised progesterone as the first choice for combining with oestrogen, for protection of the womb lining in women who still have their uterus.[278]

When compared with medroxyprogesterone acetate (the progestin used in the WHI), micronised progesterone has been shown to improve quality of life, by significantly improving vasomotor symptoms, anxiety, and depressive symptoms;[279] and improving sleep.[280] In addition to improving menopausal symptoms, a small study, published in 1989, showed that micronised oestradiol and progesterone resulted in decreased total cholesterol and increased HDL (good) cholesterol, with minimal side effects.[281] Recent evidence suggests that micronised progesterone can also reduce the risk of blood clots and stroke, as explained in the previous chapter.[282]

TESTOSTERONE

Testogel and Testim are examples of testosterone gels, which are available for men for treating hypogonadism. These preparations are sometimes used off label on a private prescription for postmenopausal women (rarely in premenopausal women), although only a small amount is used to account for the fact that testosterone levels are much higher in men than in women. Another, and possibly more accurate, way to provide testosterone is via a compounding pharmacy (see below), as the correct dose can be delivered by a measured pump and the dose can be personalised to fit the patient. The most common side effects in women are an increase in facial hair or growth of fine hair on the skin surface where the cream or gel has been applied (for this reason you will probably be advised to rotate the application to different areas of the body). Women prone to acne should be aware that this condition can reoccur when using testosterone. Hypersexuality and an increase in aggressive behaviour have been reported and in very rare cases an increase in the size of the clitoris. However, the side effects if taken in the correct dose and kept within normal physiological levels are few and you will be closely monitored by your doctor if this is prescribed for you.

COMPOUNDING PHARMACIES

Compounded hormone therapies are commonly prescribed, often in combination with some testing for hormone levels, although there is controversy about their safety and efficacy. This is because there are very few studies examining safety and efficacy, and which compare compounded hormones with FDA-regulated hormones. It should be noted however that compounding pharmacies use some of the same ingredients that are made into FDA-approved products, but the finished products are not FDA-approved or regulated. They are however strictly regulated.

The compounded oestrogen formulations most frequently prescribed contain oestradiol, oestrone, and oestriol in varying percentages, according to individual needs. Two common formulations, known as bi-oestrogen (bi-est) and tri-oestorgen (tri-est) are available in oral, transdermal, and vaginal preparations:[283]

▶ Bi-est contains 80 per cent oestriol, with 20 per cent 17β-oestradiol.

▶ Tri-est contains 10 per cent oestrone, 10 per cent 17β-oestradiol, and 80 per cent oestriol.

The reason some specialists prescribe oestriol, as well as oestradiol, is because some research has suggested that oestriol could have a protective effect against breast cancer. There are two oestrogen 'receptors': ER alpha (found predominantly in breast and womb tissue), and ER beta (found predominantly in bone and blood vessels). Research has been carried out to determine which type of oestrogen binds to which receptor:[284,285]

▶ 17 beta-oestradiol binds to both ER alpha and ER beta (so can affect all cells above).

▶ Oestrone predominantly binds to ER alpha (so mainly affects cells in the womb and breast).

▶ Oestriol has the weakest binding activity for either receptor, but binds predominantly to ER beta (so mainly affects bone and blood vessels, and may have less effect on the womb and breasts).

Although this area of research is very complex, these patterns have influenced how menopause experts tailor their prescriptions for individual needs, in order to maximise benefits and minimise risks. If you are considering using compounded hormones, you must make sure your prescribing doctor has considerable experience with bioidentical hormones and a long-term relationship with the particular compounding pharmacy that they use.

Here are a few questions that you may want to ask of them:

▶ Where does the pharmacy source its chemicals? *There are a number of different companies that supply to compounding pharmacies. For example, MEDISCA is an FDA-registered supplier of pharmacy compounding products and services the North American, Australian, and international markets. All chemicals should come with a certificate of analysis, so that the compounding pharmacist can be sure of composition and purity.*

▶ What kind of equipment is used to ensure that the cream adequately penetrates through the skin and that each pump has the exact same amount of active ingredient? *This could include where the base cream comes from; if the active ingredients are micronised or not (made smaller for better absorption); and equipment that can include ointment mills, or unguators (high speed mixers).*

▶ What in-house procedures does the pharmacy follow to ensure quality? Is there a programme in place that continually tests the quality of their products?

▶ What kind of outside testing does the pharmacy do to ensure quality and what percentage of daily volume is tested in this way? *This should include how many samples (and how often) are sent, and the name of the independent company which analyses them.*

▶ Ask to see the pharmacy's certificates of analysis on the products it has tested.

▶ Is the purity of the compounded product within 10 per cent or below of the labelled strength? *The answer should, of course, be 'yes' and the certificate of analysis mentioned above should show this.*

▶ Under which organisation is the pharmacy accredited? *In the UK, the General Pharmaceutical Council (GPhC) is the independent regulator for pharmacists, pharmacy technicians and pharmacy premises. In the USA, all pharmacies and pharmacists are licensed and strictly regulated by State Boards of Pharmacy. Standards set by agencies, such as the United States Pharmacopeia (USP) and the Pharmacy Compounding Accreditation Board (PCAB) are integrated into the day-to-day practice of pharmacy compounding and are mandated by law in most states. Australia has the Pharmacy Board of Australia.*

To help you further, here is a brief summary of the pros and cons of using compounded hormones:

Pros

▶ Hormones can be prescribed in doses and preparations that are not routinely available. For example, oestriol is not available in the UK except from compounding pharmacists.

▶ Some regulated hormonal preparations may not be suitable for you. For example, micronised progesterone is not suitable for those with a soya allergy but it is possible to compound micronised progesterone without any soya involved.

▶ Most doctors who specialise in bioidentical hormones base their prescription on individual assessments of a woman's hormone levels and then personalised doses can be prescribed. In other words, it is not a 'one size fits all' approach.

Cons

▶ There is no proof that compounded hormones have fewer side effects or are more effective than licensed and FDA-approved hormone preparations.

▶ The use of 'custom-compounded bioidentical hormone therapy' is not recommended by the major menopause societies[286] due to lack of data for efficacy and safety. However, evidence is lacking mainly because very few studies have been performed to assess this.

Chapter 8 summary

In the last two chapters, we have given you a lot of information to digest. We hope the summary below will help you to decide if HRT is right for you:

▶ HRT is the most effective treatment for hot flushes, night sweats, and associated sleep disturbances.

▶ The decision to take, or not take, HRT should be a joint one between you and your doctor after benefits and risks have been made clear.

▶ FDA-approved/regulated bioidentical hormones should not be confused with compounded bioidentical hormones and may have some advantages over non-identical varieties of HRT, according to the British Menopause Society and other experts.

▶ Compounded bioidentical hormones are not recommended by the major menopause societies, mainly because of the lack of studies showing safety and efficacy (very few studies have been performed to assess compounded hormones). In some cases compounded hormones may be appropriate but they must be prescribed by a specialist who is experienced in this area. For example, if you have a soya allergy and want to take micronised progesterone or want to take oestriol, in addition to oestradiol.

▶ Oestrogen taken alone is only appropriate in women after hysterectomy. If a woman still has her uterus, a progestogen (either micronised progesterone or a progestin) must be prescribed in addition to oestrogen to protect the womb lining.

▶ The dose and duration of HRT should be worked out on an individual basis and should be consistent with treatment goals and safety issues.

▶ HRT should be prescribed at the lowest possible dose for the shortest time possible, except in POI or early menopause. The dose can be increased gradually until symptom relief is achieved.

▶ Women with POI should be encouraged to use HRT at least until the average age of the natural menopause (51).

▶ Women taking HRT should have at least an annual check-up to include an update of medical and family history, a reappraisal of individual risks and benefits, and a physical examination if considered appropriate.

▶ When only vaginal symptoms are present, low-dose vaginal oestrogen is the most effective treatment.

▶ HRT is not recommended for the routine management of long-term health problems or chronic disease.

▶ Starting HRT at the early onset of menopause and carrying on for a few years apparently carries little risk in healthy women.

▶ If HRT is to be started over age 60, the lowest possible does should be used and the transdermal route is preferable.

▶ If you have underlying medical conditions, such as higher risk of blood clots, stroke, gallbladder disease, high triglyceride levels, or high blood pressure (or family history of these conditions), transdermal HRT may be best for you. Transdermal oestrogen and implants are not associated with an increased risk of VTE.

▶ HRT is effective for preventing osteoporotic fractures although it should not be used solely for this purpose, in the absence of menopausal symptoms (other medications specific for this purpose should be discussed with your doctor).

In the next chapter, we will discuss non-hormonal treatments that may be suitable for you, if HRT is not an option, and tests that your doctor may recommend.

Chapter 9

MEDICAL MANAGEMENT

Not all women need medical help or advice leading up to, during, or after the menopause. A lucky few have no symptoms at all. Some have mild symptoms and just let them pass, whilst others find that making dietary or lifestyle changes is enough to alleviate their symptoms. However, if the range of nutritional and lifestyle approaches detailed in Chapters 2 to 6 have not helped to improve or alleviate your symptoms, this chapter explains your options if you cannot, or do not want to, take HRT, for example, if you have a personal or family history of breast cancer, endometrial cancer, or heart disease. In such cases, your doctor may recommend one of the following prescription drugs. Please be aware that all medications have side effects and the decision to take them should therefore be considered carefully. The choices broadly fall into two categories: therapies with hormone-like actions and those with non-hormonal actions.

Therapies with hormone-like actions

Tibolone

Tibolone is a synthetic steroid which has similar effects to continuously combined oestrogen and progestin HRT. Because it has hormone-like actions, it has a similar risk profile to HRT. As with conventional HRT, it has both benefits and risks.

Benefits

▶ Symptom relief – alleviates hot flushes and night sweats; has favourable effects on mood; treats vaginal/ urinary tract symptoms; and may also improve sexual interest and responsiveness.

▶ Osteoporosis prevention – prevents bone loss and has been shown to reduce fractures in older women, aged 60–85. In the same study, the risks for both breast and colon cancer were also reduced with tibolone compared with placebo. There were no differences in the risk of either heart disease or blood clots between the tibolone and placebo groups.[287]

▶ In a review in 2009, tibolone was found to reduce the risk of breast cancer in middle-aged women who had not had breast cancer before.[288] A study using the General Practice Research Database found no significant increase in risk.[289] *Note*: other studies have shown tibolone to increase breast cancer and also cause relapse in breast cancer survivors (see below).

▶ Tibolone does not generally cause breast tenderness, unlike some forms of HRT. It is uncommon for women using tibolone to experience breast tenderness (unlike standard oral oestrogen–progestin therapy HRT).

Risks

▶ Tibolone should not be prescribed with other hormone therapy and should not be taken if you have breast cancer, or have had it in the past.[290]

▶ Vaginal bleeding or spotting may occur during the first months of treatment, although this is uncommon. Also, some women report fluid retention and mild weight gain.

▶ Tibolone increases the risk of stroke.[291] In the study quoted above, involving women aged 60–85 with osteoporosis, tibolone increased the risk of stroke after 34 months of treatment and was stopped early for this reason in February 2006, at the recommendation of the data and safety monitoring board.[292] The risk increased from the first year of treatment. The baseline risk of stroke is strongly age-dependent, and so the risk with tibolone increases with older age.

▶ Most studies show an increased risk of having endometrial cancer diagnosed in tibolone users, with the risk increasing with longer duration of use. In the study above,[293] tibolone users were diagnosed with four additional cases of endometrial cancer compared with placebo users, after 2.7 years of treatment. However, the fact that these women were being screened for endometrial cancer may, at least in part, account for the increased diagnosis.

▶ As with conventional HRT, some studies have shown a similar increased risk of breast cancer in tibolone users.[294,295] The risk increased with longer duration of use but returned to baseline within a few years of stopping treatment, meaning that the risk became the same as a woman, of the same age, who never took

Tibolone. However, not all studies show an increased risk. In a study of older women aged 60–85, with osteoporosis, the risk for breast cancer was reduced with tibolone compared with the placebo group, after 34 months of treatment.[296] It is not fully understood why this result contradicted other studies.

Take home message for tibolone

▶ In younger women, the risk profile of tibolone is broadly similar to that for conventional HRT (oestrogen only, or oestrogen and progestin combined), with a possible increased risk of breast cancer to consider.

▶ For women older than about 60, the risks associated with tibolone start to outweigh the benefits because of the increased risk of stroke.

▶ If you are considering taking tibolone or HRT, you should discuss your personal and family history with your doctor so that they can assist you in making a decision. Other options may be more suitable for you.

Selective oestrogen receptor modulators

Selective oestrogen receptor modulators (SERMs) are a group of medicines, which can be 'selective', depending on the condition they are prescribed for. This means SERMs can either block oestrogen's negative action (such as in a breast cancer patient), or activate oestrogen's positive action in other cells, such as bone cells. This is possible because oestrogen receptors have a slightly different structure, depending on the kind of cell it is in. For example, in breast tissue, SERMs work by blocking the oestrogen receptors, so that oestrogen cannot attach to the cell. If oestrogen isn't attached to a breast cell, the cell doesn't receive oestrogen's signals to grow and multiply.

Benefits

▶ Breast cancer – tamoxifen is probably one of the most recognised SERMs, used to treat hormone receptor-positive breast cancer. Raloxifene is another example, also used to reduce the risk of certain types of breast cancer and also for cancer treatment.[297]

▶ Fracture reduction – raloxifene produces modest increases in bone mineral density and is licensed for use in people with spine fractures. Tamoxifen has also been shown to reduce fractures.

Risks

▶ A review of studies, published in 2009, showed an increased risk of blood clots in women taking tamoxifen and raloxifene, although the risk returned to normal after discontinuation of treatment.[298]

▶ In the same review, tamoxifen increased the risk of endometrial cancer, although raloxifene did not.[299]

▶ If you have been prescribed tamoxifen following chemotherapy, it is important to make your doctor aware if you are still menstruating as this could impact on bone health.[300]

▶ Hot flushes have been known to increase with raloxifene and tamoxifen treatment and leg cramps have been reported by women taking raloxifene.[301]

Two relatively new SERMs, approved in the USA and Europe, are ospemifene and bazedoxifene (BZA). Ospemifene is approved for the treatment of pain during intercourse. The SERM bazedoxifene (BZA), is approved as a treatment for osteoporosis and has also recently been combined with CEE (conjugated equine estrogens), to form what is called a 'tissue-selective oestrogen receptor complex' (as reported in the previous chapter, some experts believe CEEs are no longer appropriate). BZA is considered a promising replacement to the progestin used in hormonal treatment and this combination can be used to provide symptom relief and reduce fracture risks. It has similar risks to HRT, such as risk of blood clots, stroke, and gallstones. However, because BZA blocks oestrogen from reaching certain cells in the lining of the uterus and breast tissue, it is thought to protect against overgrowth and risk of cancer of the breast and uterus. One example is Duavee, which is intended only for postmenopausal women who still have a uterus. Like other products containing oestrogen, Duavee should be used for the shortest duration consistent with treatment goals and risks for the individual woman.

Take home message for SERMs

Benefits of SERMs include reduced risk of breast cancer and bone fractures, although this has to be balanced against the increased risks of blood clots and endometrial cancer. As with HRT, the balance of benefits and risks will very much depend on your own individual risk–benefit profile, based on personal and family history, and your symptoms.

Non-hormonal options

Non-hormonal treatments that have been tested in studies for their effects on hot flushes include selective serotonin reuptake inhibitors, serotonin–norepinephrine reuptake inhibitors, gabapentin, and clonidine.

Selective serotonin reuptake inhibitors (SSRIs)

Selective serotonin reuptake inhibitors (SSRIs) are a type of antidepressant medication, used mainly to treat depression and anxiety, which are sometimes prescribed to treat hot flushes. They work by increasing levels of serotonin (which is a neurotransmitter) in the brain.

SSRIs that have been tested in studies and shown to improve hot flushes include paroxetine,[302] fluoxetine,[303] and escitalopram.[304] The relief of symptoms usually occurs within one to two weeks, more rapidly than the relief of depressive symptoms, which can take six weeks or longer. However, these studies were short, lasting only a few weeks. In contrast, a nine-month study in 2005 of citalopram and fluoxetine showed no benefit for hot flushes, although those in the citalopram group did find that insomnia improved.[305] When results from this and other studies were pooled and analysed in 2014, the authors concluded that 'all other SSRIs (escitalopram, citalopram and fluoxetine) were more effective than placebo' at decreasing hot flush frequency and severity over a four to eight week period, although results suggest that escitalopram may be more effective than other SSRIs. Reported side-effects included nausea, drowsiness, sleep disturbance, dizziness/vertigo, and decreased libido.[306] However, use of the lowest dose may minimise these effects.

Take home message for SSRIs

Although not as effective as HRT, some SSRIs have been shown to improve the severity and frequency of hot flushes and appear to be a reasonable alternative to HRT in women who cannot take HRT or are concerned about the long-term effects. Results of studies collectively seem to suggest that escitalopram may be more effective than other SSRIs. The use of SSRIs may be limited by side effects (nausea, drowsiness, sleep disturbance, dizziness/vertigo, and decreased libido) in some women.

Serotonin–norepinephrine reuptake inhibitors

Serotonin–norepinephrine reuptake inhibitors (SNRIs), also antidepressants, work in a similar way to SSRIs, although they also increase levels of norepinephrine, or noradrenalin, in the brain (norepinephrine and noradrenalin are the same chemical/hormone, except noradrenalin is derived from Latin, and norepinephrine is derived from Greek).

Venlafaxine reduced the severity of hot flushes in a trial of 229 women. After four weeks of treatment, hot flush scores were reduced by 27 per cent (placebo), 37 per cent (37.5mg), and 61 per cent (75mg and 150mg), although frequencies of some side effects, such as dry mouth, decreased appetite, nausea, and constipation, were higher in the 75mg and 150mg groups than in the placebo group.[307] Nausea is the most common side effect,[308] which may cause some women to stop taking it before benefits have been experienced.

Take home message for SNRIs

As with SSRIs, SNRIs are not as effective as HRT in reducing the frequency and severity of hot flushes, and its side effects (especially nausea) may lead to withdrawal from therapy before maximum symptom relief has been achieved. Venlafaxine at a dose of 37.5mg seems preferable, since side effects were worse at higher doses.

Gabapentin

Gabapentin is an anti-epileptic drug, also prescribed for the treatment of pain, and there is evidence that it is effective for reducing hot flushes at doses of 300–900mg daily.[309]

In one trial, 197 menopausal women aged 45–65 years were randomly split into two groups to receive either gabapentin (900mg daily) or placebo for four weeks. In the gabapentin group, hot flush scores decreased by

51 per cent as compared with a 26 per cent reduction in the placebo group. These women reported greater dizziness, unsteadiness, and drowsiness at week one compared with those taking placebo; however, these symptoms improved by week two and returned to initial levels by week four.[310]

A review of studies in 2009, comparing gabapentin and placebo, reported reductions of 20 to 30 per cent in the frequency and severity of hot flushes with gabapentin. However, the side effects of dizziness, unsteadiness, fatigue, and drowsiness resulted in a higher dropout rate in the gabapentin-treated patients than in the placebo group.[311] Some experts believe its use is limited by these side effects, particularly at high doses, and suggest a stepwise increase in dosage by 300mg per week up to a maximum of 1.2g to try to minimise side effects.[312]

Take home message for gabapentin

Gabapentin appears to be effective for reducing hot flushes at doses of 300–900mg/day, although not without side effects. However, these effects may reduce, or even disappear, over time.

Clonidine

Clonidine is a drug used to treat high blood pressure, which is sometimes prescribed for the management of hot flushes in women. However, studies of clonidine for this purpose have been small and most show no benefit over placebo. When the results of studies are pooled and analysed, clonidine shows a marginal benefit over dummy pills.[313]

A comprehensive review in 2010 concluded that SSRIs, SNRIs, Gabapentin and Clonidine all reduced the number and severity of hot flushes, although it was not possible to say if some treatments are better than others. Also, side effects were inconsistently reported in the studies.[314]

A dose of 50 to 75 micrograms twice a day may be effective in some women, although the effect is modest. The most common side effect, dry mouth, is dose-related.[315] Other reported side effects are sedation, depression, dizziness, constipation, and fluid retention. It may take two to four weeks for clonidine to be fully effective. Transdermal clonidine may however be more effective than taking it orally, as one trial showed it to be effective at reducing the frequency of hot flushes.

Take home message for clonidine

Although clonidine is not as effective as HRT at reducing hot flushes, clonidine may be an option if HRT is not suitable for you. It may reduce the number and severity of hot flushes if taken for two to four weeks.

Vaginal lubricants

If vaginal dryness is your only concern, a vaginal lubricant or moisturiser may be effective to provide temporary relief from dryness and related pain during sex. A wide variety of lubricants are commercially available and can be either water-based, silicone-based, or oil-based. Water-based lubricants, such as K-Y Jelly, have the advantage of being non-staining. Oil-based lubricants (such as petroleum jelly and baby oil) should be avoided, as they can cause vaginal irritation and are associated with high rates of latex condom breakage that can lead to sexually transmitted infections. Polyurethane condoms do not break with oil-based lubricants.

Vaginal moisturisers

Like lubricants, vaginal moisturisers, such as Replens, reduce the painful friction that sex can cause as a result of vaginal dryness. Moisturisers, unlike lubricants, are absorbed into the skin and cling to the vaginal lining in a way that mimics natural secretions. Another difference is that moisturisers are applied regularly, not just before sex, and their effects are more long-term, lasting up to three or four days. Some moisturisers have an applicator to help place the product into the vagina. Because moisturisers maintain vaginal moisture and acidity, they are particularly appropriate for midlife women who are bothered by symptoms of vaginal dryness (such as irritation and burning) that are experienced generally, not only when engaging in sexual activity. For both moisturisers and lubricants, you may need to experiment with several products to find the one that's best for you. A few examples are Replens, Sylk, Yes, Regelle and Pjur.[316]

Osteoporosis medications

Before you read the following, you should read about the nutritional and lifestyle factors that can influence bone health in Chapters 2 to 6. If you have been diagnosed with osteopenia (the precursor to osteoporosis), it may be possible to improve your bone mineral density (BMD) by doing regular, weight-bearing exercise and taking specific supplements for bone health. Even with a diagnosis of osteoporosis (if you haven't already had a fracture), it may be possible to delay treatment. As explained in the previous chapter, HRT may be recommended for osteoporosis prevention or treatment if you have menopausal symptoms and/or have experienced early menopause (before the age of 51). However, if you don't have menopausal symptoms, HRT will not be recommended purely for osteoporosis, since options other than HRT are considered effective.[317]

Bishosphonates

Bisphosphonates (BPs), including Fosamax (alendronate) and Actonel (risedronate), are medications that are prescribed for both prevention and treatment of postmenopausal osteoporosis.

HOW THEY WORK

Cells that clear old bone to make way for new bone are called osteoclast cells; and the cells that are involved in the bone-building process are called osteoblasts. BPs work by affecting the activity of the osteoclast cells, which slows down the bone-clearing process. A wealth of information from clinical trials has shown that BPs are effective at limiting the loss of bone mass, deterioration of bone structure, and increased fracture risk that occur with ageing. The best effects typically occur within three months of starting oral BPs, although effects are seen faster after intravenous (IV) BP therapy. However, more recently, concerns have been raised regarding the optimal duration of use and the long-term effects on bone quality, as explained below.

Note: It is very important to ensure adequate calcium and vitamin D intake before and during therapy with BPs.

SIDE EFFECTS

The most common side effects are related to the gastrointestinal (GI) tract and include nausea, indigestion, heartburn, vomiting, abdominal pain, and inflammation of the stomach lining (gastritis). Patients are counselled to take the medication with a full glass of water on an empty stomach in the morning. They must then stay fully upright (sitting, standing, or walking) for at least 30 minutes and must not lie down until after their first food of the day. Failing to do so, may lead to a condition called erosive esophagitis (irritation or inflammation of the oesophagus). Some patients who receive IV BPs (approximately one in three), may experience fever and other flu-like symptoms, usually lasting 24 to 72 hours. However, clinical trials of IV zoledronic acid suggest that although this may happen with the first infusion, the incidence declines with subsequent infusions (1 in 15 patients with a second infusion and 1 in 35 patients with a third infusion). Although much less common with oral BPs, this reaction may occur, especially after initiation of therapy. Treatment with paracetamol may ameliorate these symptoms, which otherwise spontaneously resolve.

It has recently been reported that the severe suppression of bone turnover could actually lead to more fractures if used long-term. In particular, the long-term use of BPs has been linked to the occurrence of atypical femoral fractures (AFFs). It is not fully understood why this happens, although it has been suggested that the long-term, continual suppression of the bone-clearing process, which in turn can alter the bone quality and fracture repair process, could lead to the development of AFFs.[318–323] Studies indicate that the absolute incidence of AFFs is relatively low (estimated between 0.3 and 11 per 100,000 person years), but there does appear to be an association between long-term BP use (5 years or more) and the incidence of AFFs. The US Food and Drug Administration published a systematic review of trials in 2011 evaluating the effects of continuous versus time-limited drug treatment. They state that: 'The observational studies have mostly shown an increased risk of atypical fractures among bisphosphonate users compared to non-users although the incidence rates are very low in both groups. The evidence with regard to long-term exposure is conflicting.'[324]

This risk may be reduced by taking a 'medication holiday'. Because BPs accumulate in bone, they create a reservoir leading to continued release from bone for months or years after treatment is stopped. Studies with risedronate and alendronate suggest that if treatment is stopped after three to five years, there is persisting anti-fracture efficacy, at least for one to two years. Some experts recommend a drug holiday after five to ten years of BP treatment. The duration of treatment and length of the holiday are based on fracture risk and the properties of the BP taken. In an article published in 2010, Watts and Diab suggest:

Patients at mild risk might stop treatment after 5 yr and remain off as long as bone mineral density is stable and no fractures occur. Higher risk patients should be treated for 10 yr, have a holiday of no more than a year or two, and perhaps be on a non-bisphosphonate treatment during that time.[325]

Studies of alendronate and zoledronic acid also showed that residual fracture benefits were seen in patients who discontinued treatment for three to five years after an initial three- to five-year treatment period. If you are, or have been, prescribed BPs, you should discuss this with your doctor and/or have your BMD and fracture risk assessed regularly to determine whether treatment could be stopped, or should be reinitiated.

Is osteoporosis over diagnosed?

Before the late 1980s, osteoporosis was diagnosed after a bone fracture. The advent of dual energy x-ray absorptiometry (DXA) made it possible to measure BMD and allowed earlier diagnosis. In 1994 a World Health Organisation (WHO) Study Group published the first diagnostic criteria for osteoporosis.

The scan measures your BMD and compares it to the ideal or peak BMD of a healthy 30-year-old adult, and gives you a score, called a T-score. A score of 0 means your BMD is equal to the norm for a healthy young adult. Differences between your BMD and that of the healthy young adult norm are measured in units called standard deviations (SDs). The more SDs below 0, indicated as negative numbers, the lower your BMD and the higher your risk of fracture. Put simply:

- A T-score between +1 and −1 is considered normal or healthy.

- A T-score between −1 and −2.5 indicates low bone mass, although not low enough to be diagnosed with osteoporosis. This is called osteopenia.

- A T-score of −2.5 or lower indicates that you have osteoporosis. The greater the negative number, the more severe the osteoporosis.

According to a recent meta-analysis, published in the prestigious *British Medical Journal*, there is evidence of over-diagnosis of osteoporosis, which can cause psychological harm, in addition to the possible adverse effects of medications, as described above. Women found to have low BMD, and also being labelled as at risk of fracture, were more likely to take measures to prevent fractures than those with normal density. They also became more fearful of falling and were more likely to limit their activities to avoid falling. The authors argue that fractures have more to do with impaired balance than bone fragility and that fewer than one in three hip fractures are attributable to bone fragility, with most hip fractures occurring in people without osteoporosis. They say that the question, 'do you have impaired balance?' can predict about 40 per cent of all hip fractures, whereas osteoporosis predicts less than 30 per cent. They reviewed the evidence for BPs, which included 33 randomised controlled trials (RCTs) of sufficient duration to expect a preventive effect on hip fractures (one year or more). Their results indicated that 175 postmenopausal women with bone fragility must be treated for about three years to prevent one hip fracture and the authors concluded that those most prone to hip fractures may not benefit from treatment with bisphosphonates. They challenge the current medical approach that assumes that bone fragility, assessed by BMD or fracture risk calculators, predicts hip fracture and that subsequent drug treatment prevents fractures.[326]

Other osteoporosis treatments

Other treatments for postmenopausal osteoporosis include parathyroid hormone (PTH), strontium ranelate, and denosumab, although we will not cover these in detail as BPs are the first-line therapy. Evidence from bone-quality studies suggest that women, aged 60–65 years, with very low BMD T-scores (high risk) may benefit from PTH as primary therapy to improve and build bone and that PTH treatment with bisphosphonates will maintain improvements in bone quality and reduce the risk of fracture.[327] Your doctor or specialist will decide which is the best treatment for you based on your individual assessments.

Take home message for osteoporosis medications

▶ Studies have shown that bisphosphonates (BPs) are effective for both prevention and treatment of postmenopausal osteoporosis. They limit the loss of bone mass, deterioration of bone structure, and increased fracture risk that occur with ageing, by slowing down the bone-clearing process.

▶ Possible side effects of BPs include nausea, dyspepsia, abdominal pain, gastritis, and severe suppression of bone turnover, which can lead to atypical femoral fractures (AFFs).

▶ Because BPs accumulate in bone, their effects can continue for months or years after treatment is stopped. Treatment should therefore be continually reviewed and a 'treatment holiday' may be taken if considered appropriate.

▶ Other osteoporosis treatments include parathyroid hormone (PTH), strontium ranelate, and denosumab, although these are generally used in either high-risk patients, or in those patients for whom BPs are not suitable.

▶ Please read Chapters 2, 3, and 6 for details on how nutrition and lifestyle changes can be effective for improving bone health.

Tests your doctor may recommend

In addition to hormone levels, your doctor may want to measure cholesterol and other fats in the blood (to assess heart health), and also your liver function / health, particularly if prescribing oral medications (as they have to first pass through the liver).

Many women have asked if hormone level tests are reliable. As explained in Chapter 1, the test most often performed to determine menopausal status is FSH, although sometimes menopausal status can be determined by symptoms alone. Other hormones that may be measured include oestradiol, progesterone, testosterone, thyroid hormones, DHEA, and vitamin D, although not all doctors carry out a huge array of tests as they consider symptom changes / improvements adequate to assess treatment strategies. However, some doctors and specialists rely on them and some even refuse further treatment unless certain tests are performed. There is some controversy as to which are the most accurate and meaningful – no method of testing is perfect and it depends on what your doctor wishes to assess. The following section may be of benefit if you have been recommended to have any of the tests described below. However, the majority of these tests will only be recommended by a doctor/specialist if they are considered necessary, for example based on your symptoms and/or health history.

Which is more accurate, blood or saliva?

Hormones such as oestrogen, progesterone, testosterone, DHEA, and cortisol in the bloodstream are mostly (95–99 per cent) bound to carrier proteins, making them unavailable to their target tissues/receptors. It is only the unbound fraction (1–5 per cent) that is available to freely diffuse into the target tissue. Supporters of saliva testing stress that the hormone levels in saliva represent the quantity of hormone that is available to target tissue and is therefore able to exert specific effects on the body (this is called 'free' or 'unbound'). Whether blood or saliva is a better sample is a debate that rages on and has done for some years. Since no definitive conclusion has been reached, we will not go into great detail. Suffice it to say that both saliva and blood testing have their own strengths and weaknesses. The important thing is consistency and comparing like with like. For example, don't see a doctor who using saliva testing and then change to a doctor who uses blood testing as it will be impossible to compare the results.

Measuring stress hormones

Most experts agree that saliva is the best way to test stress hormones, such as cortisol. Excess cortisol can adversely affect many areas in the body, such as bone and muscle tissue, heart health, sleep, thyroid function, weight control, and our immune systems. Over time, cortisol secretion can become impaired, resulting in an inability to respond to stress. It is possible to test your cortisol levels by taking four saliva samples over a 24-hour period (one first thing in the morning, one immediately before you go to bed, and two evenly spaced in between) which can then be analysed for levels of cortisol and DHEA (this is usually done at home and sent to the lab in the post). The test can shed light on biochemical imbalances underlying many conditions and is a useful test if you suffer from high levels of stress, anxiety, depression, extreme fatigue, thyroid problems, insomnia, or difficulty balancing your blood sugar.

Thyroid tests

The thyroid gland is located in the front of the neck above your collarbone. Its main job is to manufacture the thyroid hormones that regulate metabolism and affect nearly every cell, tissue, and organ in the body. When the thyroid becomes imbalanced, which it does in approximately one in eight women, the problem can be either an underactive thyroid (hypothyroidism) or an overactive thyroid (hyperthyroidism).

Hypothyroidism

An underactive thyroid occurs when the thyroid no longer produces enough of the hormones to keep the body functioning properly. If untreated, it can lead to high cholesterol, osteoporosis, heart disease, and depression. Some symptoms of hypothyroidism are similar to symptoms reported during the menopause, including fatigue, forgetfulness, mood swings, weight gain, irregular menstrual cycles, and cold intolerance.

Hyperthyroidism

An overactive thyroid occurs when the thyroid produces too much of its hormones. Some symptoms of hyperthyroidism can also mimic those of the menopause transition, including hot flushes, heat intolerance, palpitations, tachycardia (persistent rapid heartbeat), and insomnia. The most common signs of hyperthyroidism are unplanned weight loss, exophthalmos (bulging eyes) and goitre (an enlarged thyroid gland), although thyroid goitre may be associated with both hypo- and hyper-thyroidism.

Your doctor can test for both these conditions if s/he believes this could be an issue for you. Most mainstream doctors will only test levels of thyroid-stimulating hormone (TSH) and T4. Testing for free (unbound) T3, and T4 are usually only done privately.

What do urine tests reveal?

Urine tests, or urinalysis, are most commonly used to detect a wide range of disorders, such as urinary tract infection, kidney disease, and diabetes. Urine testing is non-invasive and convenient, as samples can be taken in the comfort of your own home.

Urine testing today can reveal a great deal about our health and body processes. For example, there has been a great deal of research on how oestrogens are processed, or metabolised, in our bodies and how these metabolites affect our health. Two particular metabolites that can be assessed are 16 alpha-hydroxyestrone (16 alpha-OHE1) and 2-hydroxyestrogen (2-OHE):

▶ Normal levels of 2-OHE imply a decreased likelihood of breast cancer, and osteopenia.

▶ Excessive levels of 2-OHE may increase the risk of osteoporosis in post-menopausal women with low oestrogen.

▶ High levels of 16 alpha-OHE1 are linked to increased risk of conditions linked to oestrogen excess such as breast cancer and lupus.

The 2-OHE:16 alpha-OHE1 ratio is the key to optimising health. High 2:16 ratios generally mean a lower risk of oestrogen-related cancers (like breast, uterine, and ovarian), whereas low 2:16 ratios mean higher risk of these same cancers.

This test is designed for both premenopausal and postmenopausal women and can also be done as a blood test. Please note that in the UK this test is only available from a specialist or nutritional therapist, who can then advise you how to improve the ratio (dietary advice and exercise).

Vaginal ultrasound scans

Your doctor may ask you to have this either annually, or bi-annually, to ensure that there is no increase in thickness of your endometrial (womb) lining, or to investigate any abnormal postmenopausal bleeding. However, not all doctors insist on this as there are medical guidelines in place, based on many studies, to ensure that oestrogen and progestogen are prescribed at the correct dosages and in the optimal balance to ensure that the womb lining is protected.

Homocysteine

What is homocysteine?

Homocysteine is an amino acid (amino acids are the building blocks of proteins), which occurs naturally in our bodies. The body produces homocysteine from the amino acid methionine, found in meat, fish, and dairy products. Foods containing methionine are transformed into homocysteine in the bloodstream (vitamins B6 (pyridoxine), B12, and folic acid are needed to make this reaction occur). Homocysteine is converted in the body to cysteine (vitamin B6 is needed for this reaction) or it can also be recycled back into methionine (by enzymes that require vitamin B12). Cysteine is an important protein in the body that has many roles. If homocysteine cannot be converted into cysteine or returned to the methionine form, levels of homocysteine in the body increase.

Why high levels can be harmful

Homocysteine levels are typically higher in men than women, and increase with age. Elevated levels are also associated with smoking, high blood pressure, elevated cholesterol level, and lack of exercise.[328] Elevated homocysteine levels have been associated with many diseases and medical conditions such as heart disease, cancer, strokes, and Alzheimer's disease, although it is still unclear whether decreasing plasma levels of homocysteine through diet or drugs may be paralleled by a reduction in cardiovascular risk.[329, 330] Among women, raised homocysteine levels are associated with decreased bone mineral density and increased risk of osteoporosis.[331] It seems that high levels are associated with certain conditions but it is not yet clear if lowering levels reduce risk. However, for now, if you have any of the risk factors for these conditions, as detailed in Chapter 1, we believe it is a good idea to get your level tested.

What should my level be?

Most clinical testing laboratories consider a homocysteine value of less than 12.0 micromoles per litre (μmol/l) as healthy, although some experts believe that levels should be even lower for optimal health. Recommended levels depend on age and gender so we will not list them all here. Your specialist will advise you if the level needs lowering.

What to do if you have a high level

The good news is that it is easy to fix with specific homocysteine-lowering nutrients. Not surprisingly, the nutrients named above (B6, B12, folate) are amongst those that are required. The form of folate used must be 'active' folate, known as 5-MTHF or 5-methyl-tetrahydrofolate. Your specialist, or nutritional therapist, can advise you what to take depending on your result.

Chapter 9 summary

▸ Although most of the alternatives to HRT are not as effective as HRT at reducing hot flushes, they may be an option for women who cannot take HRT or are concerned about the long-term effects. If you are considering taking any of these medications, you should discuss your personal and family history with your doctor so that they can assist you in making a decision. As with HRT, the balance of benefits and risks with all medications will very much depend on your personal and family history, and your symptoms.

▸ In younger women, the risks of tibolone are broadly similar to those for conventional HRT (either oestrogen only, or oestrogen and progestin combined). For women older than about 60 years, the risks associated with tibolone start to outweigh the benefits because of the increased risk of stroke.

▶ Benefits of SERMs include reduction of breast cancer and bone fractures, although this has to be balanced against the increased risks of blood clots and endometrial cancer.

▶ Some SSRIs have been shown to improve the severity and frequency of hot flushes. Results of studies collectively seem to suggest that escitalopram may be more effective than other SSRIs. However, the use of SSRIs may be limited by side effects (nausea, drowsiness, sleep disturbance, dizziness/vertigo, and decreased libido) in some women.

▶ As with SSRIs, SNRIs are not as effective as HRT in reducing the frequency and severity of hot flushes, and their side effects (especially nausea) may lead to withdrawal from therapy before maximum symptom relief has been achieved. Venlafaxine at a dose of 37.5mg seems preferable, since side effects increased at higher doses.

▶ Gabapentin appears to be effective for reducing hot flushes, although not without side effects. However, these effects may reduce, or even disappear, over time.

▶ Although clonidine is not as effective as HRT at reducing hot flushes, it may be an option if HRT is not suitable for you. It may reduce the number and severity of hot flushes if taken for two to four weeks.

▶ If you have, or are at high risk for, osteoporosis, bisphosphonates (BPs) are the first-line therapy in the absence of menopausal symptoms, or if HRT is not suitable for you. However, before embarking on a drug programme, it is very important to understand the benefits that weight-bearing exercise, together with nutrients and food supplements specific for bone health, can have in increasing bone mineral density, as explained in Chapters 2, 3 and 6.

▶ Finding out your homocysteine level is valuable, especially if you have risk factors for any of the associated diseases or health conditions.

▶ There are a variety of specialist tests that you can have relating to hormone levels, including stress hormones, although these are usually only available via a specialist or nutritional therapist. Tests that can reveal how your body is processing oestrogen are particularly helpful and worth considering if you have a history of breast cancer.

In the next and final chapter we will attempt to bring together the material presented in this book to give an overall 'state of play' in menopause research and treatment. This is to enable you to make informed decisions with regard to your healthcare and what's best for you.

Chapter 10

PULLING IT ALL TOGETHER

We realise that we have covered a huge amount of information up to this point and you may feel quite overwhelmed. In this final chapter, we will attempt to pull together all the information contained in this book to give you some specific coherent advice. We thought it may be most helpful to divide our advice based on symptom severity so that you can follow the advice most relevant to you. The 'Menopause Matters' website also offers a detailed decision tree which you may find useful when making treatment decisions. We would also advise you to consider your personal and family history and follow any additional advice for associated health issues (see below).

....

Warning

We must stress that if you are already taking medication (either for the menopause or for an entirely separate health issue) you must not stop this medication, or take supplements, without consulting your doctor or health specialist.

....

No symptoms

If you have read this book to prepare yourself for the menopause transition, you are one of the lucky few who has time to consider your options carefully. There are logical steps to take to ensure that you are best prepared to deal with any symptoms that occur. We would recommend that you read the section below for mild to moderate symptoms so that you know what to do should symptoms occur.

Mild to moderate symptoms

If your symptoms are mild to moderate, you may also have time to consider your options, depending on how bad your symptoms are. If the advice below does not help you, have a look at the 'severe' section below.

▶ Look up your symptom in the index and read the relevant sections of the book.

▶ Familiarise yourself with the basic principles for health outlined in Chapter 2. It is best to improve your diet and lifestyle first if possible before considering medications.

▶ In addition to nutritional strategies and self-help techniques, you may want to consider using psychological and behavioural therapies which have been shown to help with the management of menopausal symptoms (Chapter 4).

▶ HRT (see page 223) is the most effective treatment for hot flushes, night sweats, and associated sleep disturbances. However, if you want to try herbs first, St John's wort has been shown to reduce the frequency, duration, and severity of hot flushes and improve psychological symptoms, sleep problems, and quality of life. It has also been found to be effective for mild to moderate depression. Black cohosh is a popular herbal remedy and may benefit women during the perimenopause but there is not enough evidence at present to state this for certain.

HRT

Oestrogen taken alone is only appropriate in women after hysterectomy. If a woman still has her uterus, a progestogen must be prescribed in addition to oestrogen to protect the womb lining. Starting HRT at the early onset of menopause and carrying on for a few years apparently carries little risk in healthy women, but benefits are more likely to outweigh risks for women before the age of 60 or within ten years after menopause. If HRT is to be started over age 60, the lowest possible does should be used and the transdermal route is preferable.

Women with premature ovarian insufficiency (POI) should be encouraged to use HRT at least until the average age of the natural menopause (51 years).

FDA-approved/regulated bioidentical hormones may have some advantages over non-bioidentical varieties of HRT, according to the British Menopause Society and other experts. Guidelines from the major menopause societies around the globe all contain positive statements regarding both transdermal oestradiol and micronised progesterone. In specific clinical settings the choice of transdermal oestrogens and natural progesterone might offer significant benefits and added safety. This is because, unlike oral oestrogens, transdermal oestradiol has been shown not to increase the risk of blood clots, or stroke at doses of 50mcg or less. The transdermal route may also offer a lower risk for gallbladder disease, and possibly even breast cancer, associated with oral use of HRT.

Certainly, if you have underlying medical conditions, such as higher risk of blood clots, stroke, gallbladder disease, high triglyceride levels, or high blood pressure, transdermal HRT may be the best route of administration for you.

When only vaginal symptoms are present, low-dose, vaginal oestrogen is the most effective treatment for symptoms related to the urinary tract or sexual wellbeing, such as vaginal dryness or associated discomfort with intercourse.

Compounded hormones may be appropriate for some women in certain circumstances. For example, if you have a soya allergy and want to take micronised progesterone or want to take oestriol, in addition to oestradiol. However, they must be prescribed by a specialist who has considerable experience in this area.

Severe symptoms

If your symptoms are severe and debilitating, you may be at your wit's end, not knowing which way to turn. We would therefore offer the following advice:

1. The first thing to do is visit your doctor, if you haven't done so already, to discuss your options.

2. If you've already been prescribed medication such as HRT, or one of the other medications detailed in Chapter 9, you may need to go back if your symptoms have not improved. It might be that the dosage needs to be changed or another preparation may be more suitable for you. HRT can be prescribed at a low dose for a short time to at least tide you over until

the benefits of either nutritional strategies or other therapies kick in.

3. Hopefully your symptoms will reduce, at which time you can follow the steps for mild to moderate symptoms above, and then work with your doctor when you want to stop taking your medication. This has to be done gradually, as explained in Chapter 8.

Associated health issues

If you are concerned about bone health

If you have been diagnosed with osteoporosis, or its precursor osteopenia, or are just concerned about bone health due to your family history, follow the steps below:

1. Make sure you are doing some form of exercise, particularly weight-bearing activities such as walking or tai chi. If you can do this outdoors so much the better as you'll increase your levels vitamin D due to sunlight.

2. Also look at the food sources of calcium and vitamin D in Chapter 3 and ensure that you get plenty of these foods in your diet.

3. If you think your levels may be low, go to your doctor and ask to have your level tested (certainly if you already know you have low BMD, you should monitor your levels). If your level is low, supplement under the guidance of a health professional. If your aim is to prevent fractures, vitamin D should always be combined with calcium, although not all studies have shown a positive benefit. If you are at risk of osteoporosis and are considering supplementing calcium and vitamin D, it is best to do so as part of

a bone-building/protection formula or under the guidance of a health professional.

4. All the major menopause societies agree that HRT is effective and appropriate for the prevention of osteoporosis-related fractures in at-risk women before age 60 years, or within ten years after menopause, although HRT is not recommended for the routine management of long-term health problems or chronic disease.

5. If you don't have menopausal symptoms, bisphosphonates (BPs) will most likely be prescribed as they are effective for both prevention and treatment of postmenopausal osteoporosis. They slow down the bone-clearing process, although can have side effects (Chapter 9). However, because BPs accumulate in bone, their effects can continue for months or years after treatment is stopped, which means that you may be able to take a 'treatment holiday' if considered appropriate by your doctor.

If you are concerned about heart or cognitive health

1. Exercise – any activity is better than none so find something you enjoy and feel that you can do regularly. Keeping active and not sitting for prolonged periods is key.

2. Evening primrose oil is safe and may help with heart disease and osteoporosis, although the evidence for its effectiveness for specific menopausal symptoms is lacking.

3. Although the mechanisms by which ginseng improves health are complex and still to be completely

unravelled, some studies have seen cognitive and cardiovascular benefits.

4. There is evidence that standard-dose oestrogen-alone HRT may decrease heart disease and death from all causes in women younger than 60 years of age and within ten years of menopause. However, when oestrogen is prescribed with a progestogen no significant increase or decrease in heart disease has been found, although there is a similar trend for reducing mortality.

We sincerely hope you've found the guidance in this book helpful and we strongly advise that you discuss all treatments and strategies with your doctor or healthcare practitioner so that they can help you find the best combination of techniques for you to have the best quality of life possible.

USEFUL ADDRESSES/WEBSITES

Advertising Standards Authority (ASA)

www.asa.org.uk

rulings

www.asa.org.uk/Rulings/Adjudications.aspx

The British Association for Behavioural and Cognitive Psychotherapies (BABCP) register

www.cbtregisteruk.com/Default.aspx

BMI calculator

www.bupa.co.uk/health-information/tools-calculators/bmi-calculator or Smartphone App

British Homeopathic Association

www.britishhomeopathic.org

British Menopause Society

www.thebms.org.uk

British Psychological Society's (BPS) directory of qualified psychologists

www.bps.org.uk/bpslegacy/dcp

Complementary and Natural Healthcare Council (CNHC)

www.cnhc.org.uk

The Daisy Network

www.daisynetwork.org.uk, support group for women with POI

Drugs.com

www.drugs.com, for information on medication side effects and possible interactions with other medications/food/supplements

General Osteopathic Council

www.osteopathy.org.uk/home

General Chiropractic Council

www.gcc-uk.org

Health and Care Professions Council (HCPC)

www.hcpc-uk.org.uk

register

www.hcpc-uk.org/check/

Hypnotherapy Directory

www.hypnotherapy-directory.org.uk

International Menopause Society

www.imsociety.org

Medicines and Healthcare products Regulatory Agency

www.gov.uk/government/organisations/medicines-and-healthcare-products-regulatory-agency

for specific medicines information

www.mhra.gov.uk/spc-pil

Menopause Matters

www.menopausematters.co.uk – this site includes an interactive decision tree at www.menopausematters.co.uk/tree.php, which aims to help women explore their treatment options

TEDX (The Endocrine Disruption Exchange, Inc.)

www.endocrinedisruption.org, focuses primarily on the human health and environmental problems caused by low-dose and/or ambient exposure to chemicals that interfere with development and function, called endocrine disruptors (EDCs)

Trading Standards

www.tradingstandards.uk/advice/index.cfm

The North American Menopause Society

www.menopause.org

The Wiley Protocol

www.thewileyprotocol.com

See also: Rhythmic Living

www.rhythmicliving.org – a cautionary tale about the Wiley Protocol

Women's Health Concern

www.womens-health-concern.org

ENDNOTES

1. Harlow, S.D., Gass, M., Hall, J.E. *et al.* (2012) 'Executive summary of the Stages of Reproductive Aging Workshop + 10: Addressing the unfinished agenda of staging reproductive aging.' *Journal of Clinical Endocrinology and Metabolism 97*, 4, 1159–1168.

2. Grindler, N.M., Allsworth, J.E., Macones, G.A., Kannan, K., Roehl, K.A. and Cooper, A.R. (2015) 'Persistent organic pollutants and early menopause in U.S. women.' *PLoS One 10*, 1, e0116057.

3. Panay, N., Hamoda, H., Arya, R. and Savvas, M. (2013). 'The 2013 British Menopause Society & Women's Health Concern recommendations on hormone replacement therapy.' *Menopause International 19*, 2, 59–68.

4. Committee on Adolescent Health Care (2014) 'Primary ovarian insufficiency in adolescents and young women.' Committee Opinion No. 605. American College of Obstetricians and Gynecologists. *Obstetrics and Gynecology 123*, 193–197.

5. Genazzani, A.R., Schneider, H.P., Panay, N. and Nijland, E.A. (2006) 'The European Menopause Survey 2005: Women's perceptions on the menopause and postmenopausal hormone therapy.' *Gynecological Endocrinology 22*, 7, 369–375.

6. Freeman, E.W., Sammel, M.D. and Sanders, R.J. (2014) 'Risk of long-term hot flashes after natural menopause: Evidence from the Penn Ovarian Aging Study cohort.' *Menopause 21*, 9, 924–932.

7. Pearce, G., Thøgersen-Ntoumani, C. and Duda, J. (2014) 'Body image during the menopausal transition: A systematic scoping review.' *Body image 8*, 4, 473–489.

8. Deeks, A.A. (2003) 'Psychological aspects of menopause management.' *Best Practice & Research Clinical Endocrinology & Metabolism 17*, 1, 17–31.

9. Deeks, A.A. and McCabe, M.P. (2001) 'Menopausal stage and age and perceptions of body image.' *Psychology and Health 16*, 3, 367–379.

10. Rubinstein, H.R. and Foster, J.L.H. (2013) '"I don't know whether it is to do with age or to do with hormones and whether it is do with a stage in your life": Making sense of menopause and the body.' *Journal of Health Psychology 18*, 2, 292–307.

11. Hvas, L. (2001) 'Positive aspects of menopause: A qualitative study.' *Maturitas 39*, 1, 11–17.

12. Hvas, L. (2001) 'Positive aspects of menopause: A qualitative study.' *Maturitas 39*, 1, 11–17.

13. Hvas, L. (2006) 'Menopausal women's positive experience of growing older.' *Maturitas 54*, 3, 245–251.

14. Hvas, L. (2001) 'Positive aspects of menopause: A qualitative study.' *Maturitas 39*, 1, 11–17.

15. Brayne, S. (2011) *Sex, Meaning and the Menopause.* London: Bloomsbury Publishing.

16. Winterich, J.A. (2003) Sex, menopause, and culture sexual orientation and the meaning of menopause for women's sex lives.' *Gender & Society 17*, 4, 627–642.

17. Bloch, A. (2002) 'Self-awareness during the menopause.' *Maturitas 41*, 1, 61–68.

18. Koch, P.B., Mansfield, P.K., Thurau, D. and Carey, M. (2005) '"Feeling frumpy": The relationships between body image and sexual response changes in midlife women.' *Journal of Sex Research 42*, 3, 215–223.

19. Rubinstein, H.R. and Foster, J.L.H. (2013) '"I don't know whether it is to do with age or to do with hormones and whether it is do with a stage in your life": Making sense of menopause and the body.' *Journal of Health Psychology 18*, 2, 292–307.

20. Hvas, L. (2006) 'Menopausal women's positive experience of growing older.' *Maturitas 54*, 3, 245–251.

21. Hvas, L. (2001) 'Positive aspects of menopause: A qualitative study.' *Maturitas 39*, 1, 11–17.

22. Hvas, L. (2006) 'Menopausal women's positive experience of growing older.' *Maturitas 54*, 3, 245–251.

23. Rubinstein, H.R. and Foster, J.L.H. (2013) '"I don't know whether it is to do with age or to do with hormones and whether it is do with a stage in your life": Making sense of menopause and the body.' *Journal of Health Psychology 18*, 2, 292–307.

24. Hvas, L. (2006) 'Menopausal women's positive experience of growing older.' *Maturitas 54*, 3, 245–251.

25. Parkin, D.M., Boyd, L. and Walker, L.C. (2011) 'The fraction of cancer attributable to lifestyle and environmental factors in the UK in 2010.' *British Journal of Cancer 105*, Suppl 2:S77–81.

26. Lichtenstein, P., Holm, N.V., Verkasalo, P.K. *et al.* (2000) 'Environmental and heritable factors in the causation of cancer – analyses of cohorts of twins from Sweden, Denmark, and Finland.' *New England Journal of Medicine 343*, 2, 78–85.

27. World Cancer Research Fund (WCRF) American Institute for Cancer Research (AICR) (2007) *Food, Nutrition, Physical Activity, and the Prevention of Cancer: A Global Perspective.* Washington, DC: AICR.

28. Jonas, C.R., McCullough, M.L., Teras, L.R., Walker-Thurmond, K.A., Thun, M.J. and Calle, E.E. (2003) 'Dietary glycemic index, glycemic load, and risk of incident breast cancer in postmenopausal women.' *Cancer Epidemiology, Biomarkers and Prevention 12*, 6, 573–577.

29. American Heart Association (2015) *Healthy Workplace Food and Beverage Toolkit,* page 6. Available at www.heart.org/idc/groups/heart-public/@wcm/@fc/documents/downloadable/ucm_465693.pdf, accessed on 11 January 2016.

30. Foster-Powell, K., Holt, S.H. and Brand-Miller, J.C. (2002) 'International table of glycemic index and glycemic load values: 2002.' *American Journal of Clinical Nutrition 76*, 1, 5–56.

31. Augustin, L.S., Dal Maso, L., La Vecchia, C. *et al.* (2001) 'Dietary glycemic index and glycemic load, and breast cancer risk: A case-control study.' *Annals of Oncology 12*, 11, 1533–1538.

32. Folsom, A.R., Demissie, Z. and Harnack, L. (2003) 'Glycemic index, glycemic load, and incidence of endometrial cancer: The Iowa women's health study.' *Nutrition and Cancer 46*, 2, 119–124.

33. de Menezes, R.F., Bergmann, A. and Thuler, L.C. (2013) 'Alcohol consumption and risk of cancer: A systematic literature review.' *Asian Pacific Journal of Cancer Prevention 14*, 9, 4965–4972.

34. Bagnardi, V., Rota, M., Botteri, E. *et al.* (2013) 'Light alcohol drinking and cancer: A meta-analysis.' *Annals of Oncology 24*, 2, 301–308.

35. Cao, Y., Willett, W.C., Rimm, E.B., Stampfer, M.J. and Giovannucci, E.L. (2015) 'Light to moderate intake of alcohol, drinking patterns, and risk of cancer: Results from two prospective US cohort studies.' *British Medical Journal 351*, h4238.

36. Colborn, T., Peterson Myers, J. and Dumanoski, D. (1996) *Our Stolen Future: Are We Threatening Our Own Fertility, Intelligence, and Survival? A Scientific Detective Story.* New York: Dutton.

37. European Food Safety Authority (EFSA) Panel on Food Contact Materials, Enzymes, Flavourings and Processing Aids (CEF) (2015) 'Scientific Opinion on the risks to public health related to the presence of bisphenol A (BPA) in foodstuffs: Executive summary.' *EFSA Journal 13*, 1, 3978.

38. Panay, N. (2007) 'Integrating phytoestrogens with prescription medicines: A conservative clinical approach to vasomotor symptom management.' *Maturitas 57*, 1, 90–94.

39. Rowland, I., Faughnan, M., Hoey, L., Wähälä K., Williamson, G. and Cassidy, A. (2003) 'Bioavailability of phyto-oestrogens.' *British Journal of Nutrition 89*, Suppl 1:S45–58.

40. Messina, M., Nagata, C. and Wu, A.H. (2006) 'Estimated Asian adult soy protein and isoflavone intakes.' *Nutrition and Cancer 55*, 1, 1–12.

41. Messina, M., Nagata, C. and Wu, A.H. (2006) 'Estimated Asian adult soy protein and isoflavone intakes.' *Nutrition and Cancer 55*, 1, 1–12.

42. Chen, M.N., Lin, C.C. and Liu, C.F. (2015) 'Efficacy of phytoestrogens for menopausal symptoms: A meta-analysis and systematic review.' *Climacteric 18*, 2, 260–269.

43. Jacobs, A., Wegewitz, U., Sommerfeld, C., Grossklaus, R. and Lampen, A. (2009) 'Efficacy of isoflavones in relieving vasomotor menopausal symptoms: A systematic review.' *Molecular Nutrition and Food Research 53*, 9, 1084–1097.

44. Lethaby, A., Marjoribanks, J., Kronenberg, F., Roberts, H., Eden, J. and Brown, J. (2013) 'Phytoestrogens for menopausal vasomotor symptoms.' *Cochrane Database of Systematic Reviews 12*, CD001395.

45. Chen, M.N., Lin, C.C. and Liu, C.F. (2015) 'Efficacy of phytoestrogens for menopausal symptoms: A meta-analysis and systematic review.' *Climacteric 18*, 2, 260–269.

46. Chen, M.N., Lin, C.C. and Liu, C.F. (2015) 'Efficacy of phytoestrogens for menopausal symptoms: A meta-analysis and systematic review.' *Climacteric 18*, 2, 260–269.

47. Beecher, H.K. (1955) 'The powerful placebo.' *Journal of the American Medical Association 159*, 17, 1602–1606.

48. Wu, A.H., Yu, M.C., Tseng, C.C. and Pike, M.C. (2008) 'Epidemiology of soy exposures and breast cancer risk.' *British Journal of Cancer 98*, 1, 9–14.

49. Xu, W.H., Zheng, W., Xiang, Y.B. *et al.* (2004) 'Soya food intake and risk of endometrial cancer among Chinese women in Shanghai: Population based case-control study.' *British Medical Journal 328*, 7451, 1285.

50. Messina, M.J. and Wood, C.E. (2008) 'Soy isoflavones, estrogen therapy, and breast cancer risk: Analysis and commentary.' *Nutrition Journal 7*, 17.

51. Unfer, V., Casini, M.L., Costabile, L., Mignosa, M., Gerli, S. and Di Renzo, G.C. (2004) 'Endometrial effects of long-term treatment with phytoestrogens: A randomized, double-blind, placebo-controlled study.' *Fertility and Sterility 82*, 1, 145–148, quiz 265.

52. Quaas, A.M., Kono, N., Mack, W.J. *et al.* (2013) 'Effect of isoflavone soy protein supplementation on endometrial thickness, hyperplasia, and endometrial cancer risk in postmenopausal women: A randomized controlled trial.' *Menopause 20*, 8, 840–844.

53. Messina, M., Nagata, C. and Wu, A.H. (2006) 'Estimated Asian adult soy protein and isoflavone intakes.' *Nutrition and Cancer 55*, 1, 1–12.

54. Bitto, A., Polito, F., Atteritano, M. *et al.* (2010) 'Genistein aglycone does not affect thyroid function: Results from a three-year, randomized, double-blind, placebo-controlled trial.' *Journal of Clinical Endocrinology and Metabolism 95*, 6, 3067–3072.

55. Clarke, D.B., Bailey, V. and Lloyd, A.S. (2008) 'Determination of phytoestrogens in dietary supplements by LC-MS/MS.' *Food Additives and Contaminants. Part A, Chemistry, Analysis, Control, Exposure and Risk Assessment 25*, 5, 534–547.

56. Panay, N. (2007) 'Integrating phytoestrogens with prescription medicines: A conservative clinical approach to vasomotor symptom management.' *Maturitas 57*, 1, 90–94.

57. van de Weijer, P.H. and Barentsen, R. (2002) 'Isoflavones from red clover (Promensil) significantly reduce menopausal hot flush symptoms compared with placebo.' *Maturitas 42*, 3, 187–193.

58. Panay, N. (2007) 'Integrating phytoestrogens with prescription medicines: A conservative clinical approach to vasomotor symptom management.' *Maturitas 57*, 1, 90–94.

59. Atkinson, C., Compston, J.E., Day, N.E., Dowsett, M. and Bingham, S.A. (2004) 'The effects of phytoestrogen isoflavones on bone density in women: A double-blind, randomized, placebo-controlled trial.' *American Journal of Clinical Nutrition 79*, 2, 326–333.

60. Marini, H., Bitto, A., Altavilla, D. *et al.* (2008) 'Breast safety and efficacy of genistein aglycone for postmenopausal bone loss: A follow-up study.' *Journal of Clinical Endocrinology and Metabolism 93*, 12, 4787–4796.

61. Terzic, M.M., Dotlic, J., Maricic, S., Mihailovic, T. and Tosic-Race, B. (2009) 'Influence of red clover-derived isoflavones on serum lipid profile in postmenopausal women.' *Journal of Obstetrics and Gynaecology Research 35*, 6, 1091–1095.

62. Nestel, P.J., Pomeroy, S., Kay, S. *et al.* (1999) 'Isoflavones from red clover improve systemic arterial compliance but not plasma lipids in menopausal women.' *Journal of Clinical Endocrinology and Metabolism 84*, 3, 895–898.

63. Lipovac, M., Chedraui, P., Gruenhut, C., Gocan, A., Stammler, M. and Imhof, M. (2010) 'Improvement of postmenopausal depressive and anxiety symptoms after treatment with isoflavones derived from red clover extracts.' *Maturitas 65*, 3, 258–261.

64. Atkinson, C., Warren, R.M., Sala, E. *et al.* (2004) 'Red-clover-derived isoflavones and mammographic breast density: A double-blind, randomized, placebo-controlled trial [ISRCTN42940165].' *Breast Cancer Research 6, 3*, R170–179.

65. Marini, H., Bitto, A., Altavilla, D. *et al.* (2008) 'Breast safety and efficacy of genistein aglycone for postmenopausal bone loss: A follow-up study.' *Journal of Clinical Endocrinology and Metabolism 93*, 12, 4787–4796.

66. Panay, N., Hamoda, H., Arya, R. and Savvas, M. (2013) 'The 2013 British Menopause Society & Women's Health Concern recommendations on hormone replacement therapy.' *Menopause International 19*, 2, 59–68.

67. Carmignani, L.O., Pedro, A.O., Costa-Paiva, L.H. and Pinto-Neto, A.M. (2010) 'The effect of dietary soy supplementation compared to estrogen and placebo on menopausal symptoms: A randomized controlled trial.' *Maturitas 67*, 3, 262–269.

68. Abrahamsen, B., Masud, T., Avenell, A., Anderson, F. *et al.*(2010) 'Patient level pooled analysis of 68 500 patients from seven major vitamin D fracture trials in US and Europe.' *British Medical Journal 340*, b5463.

69. Bolland, M.J., Grey, A., Avenell, A., Gamble, G.D. and Reid, I.R. (2011) 'Calcium supplements with or without vitamin D and risk of cardiovascular events: Reanalysis of the Women's Health Initiative limited access dataset and meta-analysis.' *British Medical Journal 342*, d2040.

70. Reid, I.R. (2014) 'Should we prescribe calcium supplements for osteoporosis prevention?' *Journal of Bone Metabolism 21*, 1, 21–28.

71. Reid, I.R. (2014) 'Should we prescribe calcium supplements for osteoporosis prevention?' *Journal of Bone Metabolism 21*, 1, 21–28.

72. Reid, I.R. and Bolland, M.J. (2014) 'Skeletal and nonskeletal effects of vitamin D: Is vitamin D a tonic for bone and other tissues?' *Osteoporosis International 25*, 10, 2347–2357.

73. Bischoff-Ferrari, H.A. (2008) 'Optimal serum 25-hydroxyvitamin D levels for multiple health outcomes.' *Advances in Experimental Medicine and Biology 624*, 55–71.

74. Calder, P.C. (2012) 'Mechanisms of action of (n-3) fatty acids.' *Journal of Nutrition 142*, 3, 592s–599s.

75. Farzaneh, F., Fatehi, S., Sohrabi, M.-R. and Alizadeh, K. (2013) 'The effect of oral evening primrose oil on menopausal hot flashes: A randomized clinical trial.' *Archives of Gynecology and Obstetrics 288*, 5, 1075–1079.

76. Chenoy, R., Hussain, S., Tayob, Y., O'Brien, P.M.S., Moss, M.Y. and Morse, P.F. (1994) 'Effect of oral gamolenic acid from evening primrose oil on menopausal flushing.' *British Medical Journal 308*, 6927, 501–503.

77. Posadzki, P., Lee, M.S., Moon, T.W., Choi, T.Y., Park, T.Y. and Ernst, E. (2013) 'Prevalence of complementary and alternative medicine (CAM) use by menopausal women: A systematic review of surveys.' *Maturitas 75*, 1, 34–43.

78. Borrelli, F. and Ernst, E. (2008) 'Black cohosh (Cimicifuga racemosa) for menopausal symptoms: A systematic review of its efficacy.' *Pharmacological Research 58*, 1, 8–14.

79. Leach, M.J. and Moore, V. (2012) 'Black cohosh (Cimicifuga spp.) for menopausal symptoms.' *Cochrane Database of Systematic Reviews 9*.

80. Beer, A.M., Osmers, R., Schnitker, J., Bai, W., Mueck, A.O. and Meden, H. (2013) 'Efficacy of black cohosh (Cimicifuga racemosa) medicines for treatment of menopausal symptoms: Comments on major statements of the Cochrane

Collaboration report 2012 "black cohosh (Cimicifuga spp.) for menopausal symptoms (review)".' *Gynecology and Endocrinology 29*, 12, 1022–1025.

81. Teschke, R., Bahre, R., Genthner, A., Fuchs, J., Schmidt-Taenzer, W. and Wolff, A. (2009) 'Suspected black cohosh hepatotoxicity: Challenges and pitfalls of causality assessment.' *Maturitas 63*, 4, 302–314.

82. Naser, B., Schnitker, J., Minkin, M.J., de Arriba, S.G., Nolte, K.-U. and Osmers, R. (2011) 'Suspected black cohosh hepatotoxicity: No evidence by meta-analysis of randomized controlled clinical trials for isopropanolic black cohosh extract.' *Menopause 18*, 4, 366–375.

83. Firenzuoli, F., Gori, L. and Roberti di Sarsina, P. (2011) 'Black cohosh hepatic safety: Follow-up of 107 patients consuming a special cimicifuga racemosa rhizome herbal extract and review of literature.' *Evidence-Based Complementary and Alternative Medicine 2011*. doi:10.1093/ecam/nen009.

84. Abdali, K., Khajehei, M. and Tabatabaee, H.R. (2010) 'Effect of St John's wort on severity, frequency, and duration of hot flashes in premenopausal, perimenopausal and postmenopausal women: A randomized, double-blind, placebo-controlled study.' *Menopause 17*, 2, 326–331.

85. Grube, B., Walper, A. and Wheatley, D. (1999) 'St. John's Wort extract: Efficacy for menopausal symptoms of psychological origin.' *Advances in Therapy 16*, 4, 177–186.

86. Al-Akoum, M., Maunsell, E., Verreault, R., Provencher, L., Otis, H. and Dodin, S. (2009) 'Effects of Hypericum perforatum (St. John's wort) on hot flashes and quality of life in perimenopausal women: A randomized pilot trial.' *Menopause 16*, 2, 307–314.

87. Uebelhack, R., Blohmer, J.U., Graubaum, H.J., Busch, R., Gruenwald, J. and Wernecke, K.D. (2006) 'Black cohosh and St. John's wort for climacteric complaints: A randomized trial.' *Obstetrics and Gynecology 107*, 2 Pt 1, 247–255.

88. Qi, L.-W., Wang, C.-Z. and Yuan, C.-S. (2011) 'Ginsenosides from American ginseng: Chemical and pharmacological diversity.' *Phytochemistry 72*, 8, 689–699.

89. Geng, J., Dong, J., Ni, H. *et al.* (2010) 'Ginseng for cognition.' *Cochrane Database of Systematic Reviews 12*, Cd007769.

90. Lee, C.H. and Kim, J.-H. (2014) 'A review on the medicinal potentials of ginseng and ginsenosides on cardiovascular diseases.' *Journal of Ginseng Research 38*, 3, 161–166.

91. Kim, M.-S., Lim, H.-J., Yang, H.J., Lee, M.S., Shin, B.-C. and Ernst, E. (2013) 'Ginseng for managing menopause symptoms: A systematic review of randomized clinical trials.' *Journal of Ginseng Research 37*, 1, 30.

92. Kim, M.-S., Lim, H.-J., Yang, H.J., Lee, M.S., Shin, B.-C. and Ernst, E. (2013) 'Ginseng for managing menopause symptoms: A systematic review of randomized clinical trials.' *Journal of Ginseng Research 37*, 1, 30.

93. Kwee, S.H., Tan, H.H., Marsman, A. and Wauters, C. (2007) 'The effect of Chinese herbal medicines (CHM) on menopausal symptoms compared to hormone replacement therapy (HRT) and placebo.' *Maturitas 58*, 1, 83–90.

94. Hirata, J.D., Swiersz, L.M., Zell, B., Small, R. and Ettinger, B. (1997) 'Does dong quai have estrogenic effects in postmenopausal women? A double-blind, placebo-controlled trial.' *Fertility and Sterility 68*, 6, 981–986.

95. Kupfersztain, C., Rotem, C., Fagot, R. and Kaplan, B. (2002) 'The immediate effect of natural plant extract, Angelica sinensis and Matricaria chamomilla (Climex) for the treatment of hot flushes during menopause. A preliminary report.' *Clinical and Experimental Obstetrics and Gynecology 30*, 4, 203–206.

96. Haroon, E., Raison, C.L. and Miller, A.H. (2012) 'Psychoneuroimmunology meets neuropsychopharmacology: Translational implications of the impact of inflammation on behavior.' *Neuropsychopharmacology 37*, 1, 137–162.

97. Kiecolt-Glaser, J.K., McGuire, L., Robles, T.F. and Glaser, R. (2002) 'Psychoneuroimmunology: Psychological influences on immune function and health.' *Journal of Consulting and Clinical Psychology 70*, 3, 537.

98. Kiecolt-Glaser, J.K., McGuire, L., Robles, T.F. and Glaser, R. (2002) 'Psychoneuroimmunology and psychosomatic medicine: Back to the future.' *Psychosomatic Medicine 64*, 1, 15–28.

99. Duijts, S.F.A., van Beurden, M., Oldenburg, H.S.A. *et al.* (2012) 'Efficacy of cognitive behavioral therapy and physical exercise in alleviating treatment-induced menopausal symptoms in patients with breast cancer: Results of a randomized, controlled, multicenter trial.' *Journal of Clinical Oncology 30*, 33, 4124–4133.

100. Hofmann, S.G., Asnaani, A., Vonk, I.J.J., Sawyer, A.T. and Fang, A. (2012) 'The efficacy of cognitive behavioral therapy: A review of meta-analyses.' *Cognitive Therapy and Research 36*, 5, 427–440.

101. Newell, S.A., Sanson-Fisher, R.W. and Savolainen, N.J. (2002) 'Systematic review of psychological therapies for cancer patients: Overview and recommendations for future research.' *Journal of the National Cancer Institute 94*, 8, 558–584.

102. Gupta, P., Sturdee, D.W., Palin, S.L. *et al.* (2006) 'Menopausal symptoms in women treated for breast cancer: The prevalence and severity of symptoms and their perceived effects on quality of life.' *Climacteric 9*, 1, 49–58.

103. Hunter, M.S., Grunfeld, E.A., Mittal, S. *et al.* (2004) 'Menopausal symptoms in women with breast cancer: Prevalence and treatment preferences.' *Psycho-Oncology 13*, 11, 769–778.

104. Mann, E., Smith, M.J., Hellier, J. *et al.* (2012) 'Cognitive behavioural treatment for women who have menopausal symptoms after breast cancer treatment (MENOS 1): A randomised controlled trial.' *The Lancet Oncology 13*, 3, 309–318.

105. Ayers, B., Smith, M., Hellier, J., Mann, E. and Hunter, M.S. (2012) 'Effectiveness of group and self-help cognitive behavior therapy in reducing problematic menopausal hot flushes and night sweats (MENOS 2): A randomized controlled trial.' *Menopause 19*, 7, 749–759.

106. Gauld, A. (1992) *A History of Hypnotism*. Cambridge: Cambridge University Press.

107. Heap, M. and Aravind, K.K. (2002) *Hartland's Medical and Dental Hypnosis* (4th edn) London: Churchill Livingstone.

108. Patterson, D.R. and Jensen, M.P. (2003) 'Hypnosis and clinical pain.' *Psychological Bulletin 129*, 4, 495.

109. Hammond, D.C. (2007) 'Review of the efficacy of clinical hypnosis with headaches and migraines.' *International Journal of Clinical and Experimental Hypnosis 55*, 2, 207–219.

110. Adinolfi, B. and Gava, N. (2013) 'Controlled outcome studies of child clinical hypnosis.' *Acta Bio Medica Atenei Parmensis 84*, 2, 94–97.

111. Patterson, D.R. and Jensen, M.P. (2003) 'Hypnosis and clinical pain.' *Psychological Bulletin 129*, 4, 495.

112. Elkins, G., Marcus, J., Stearns, V. and Hasan Rajab, M. (2007) 'Pilot evaluation of hypnosis for the treatment of hot flashes in breast cancer survivors.' *Psycho-Oncology 16*, 5, 487–492.

113. Elkins, G., Marcus, J., Stearns, V. *et al.* (2008) 'Randomized trial of a hypnosis intervention for treatment of hot flashes among breast cancer survivors.' *Journal of Clinical Oncology 26*, 31, 5022–5026.

114. Elkins, G.R., Fisher, W.I., Johnson, A.K., Carpenter, J.S. and Keith, T.Z. (2013) 'Clinical hypnosis in the treatment of post-menopausal hot flashes: A randomized controlled trial.' *Menopause (New York, NY) 20*, 3, 291–298.

115. Carmody, J., Crawford, S. and Churchill L. (2006) 'A pilot study of mindfulness-based stress reduction for hot flashes.' *Menopause 13*, 5, 760–769.

116. Sharma, M. and Rush, S.E. (2014) 'Mindfulness-based stress reduction as a stress management intervention for healthy individuals a systematic review.' *Journal of Evidence-Based Complementary and Alternative Medicine 19*, 4, 271–286.

117. Innes, K.E., Selfe, T.K. and Vishnu, A. (2010) 'Mind-body therapies for menopausal symptoms: A systematic review.' *Maturitas 66*, 2, 135–149.

118. Upchurch, D.M. and Chyu, L. (2005) 'Use of complementary and alternative medicine among American women.' *Women's Health Issues 15*, 5–13.

119. Bair, Y.A., Gold, E.B., Greendale, G.A. *et al.* (2002) 'Ethnic differences in use of complementary and alternative medicine at midlife: Longitudinal results from SWAN participants.' *American Journal of Public Health 92*, 11, 1832–1840.

120. Newton, K.M., Buist, D.S.M., Keenan, N.L., Anderson, L.A. and LaCroix, A.Z. (2002) 'Use of alternative therapies for menopause symptoms: Results of a population-based survey.' *Obstetrics and Gynecology 100*, 1, 18–25.

121. Daley, A., MacArthur, C., McManus, R. *et al.* (2006) 'Factors associated with the use of complementary medicine and non-pharmacological interventions in symptomatic menopausal women.' *Climacteric 9*, 5, 336–346.

122. Upchurch, D.M. and Chyu, L. (2005) 'Use of complementary and alternative medicine among American women.' *Women's Health Issues 15*, 5–13.

123. van der Sluijs, C.P., Bensoussan, A., Liyanage, L. and Shah, S. (2007) 'Women's health during mid-life survey: The use of complementary and alternative medicine by symptomatic women transitioning through menopause in Sydney.' *Menopause 14*, 3, 397–403.

124. van der Sluijs, C.P., Bensoussan, A., Liyanage, L. and Shah, S. (2007) 'Women's health during mid-life survey: The use of complementary and alternative medicine by symptomatic women transitioning through menopause in Sydney.' *Menopause 14*, 3, 397–403.

125. Upchurch, D.M. and Chyu, L. (2005) 'Use of complementary and alternative medicine among American women.' *Women's Health Issues 15*, 5–13.

126. Daley, A., MacArthur, C., McManus, R. *et al.* (2006) 'Factors associated with the use of complementary medicine and non-pharmacological interventions in symptomatic menopausal women.' *Climacteric 9*, 5, 336–346.

127. Hill-Sakurai, L.E., Muller, J. and Thom, D.H. (2008) 'Complementary and alternative medicine for menopause: A qualitative analysis of women's decision making.' *Journal of General Internal Medicine 23*, 5, 619–622.

128. Hill-Sakurai, L.E., Muller, J. and Thom, D.H. (2008) 'Complementary and alternative medicine for menopause: A qualitative analysis of women's decision making.' *Journal of General Internal Medicine 23*, 5, 619–622.

129. Ross, A. and Thomas, S. (2010) 'The health benefits of yoga and exercise: A review of comparison studies.' *The Journal of Alternative and Complementary Medicine 16*, 1, 3–12.

130. Yang, K. (2007) 'A review of yoga programs for four leading risk factors of chronic diseases.' *Evidence-Based Complementary and Alternative Medicine 4*, 4, 487–491.

131. Cramer, H., Lauche, R., Langhorst, J. and Dobos, G. (2012) 'Effectiveness of yoga for menopausal symptoms: A systematic review and meta-analysis of randomized controlled trials.' *Evidence-Based Complementary and Alternative Medicine.* 2012. doi: 10.1155/2012/863905.

132. Pearson, P.F. (1987) *An Introduction to Acupuncture: A Practical Guide for GPs and Other Medical Personnel.* Norwell, MA: MTP Press.

133. World Health Organization (2002) *Acupuncture: Review and Analysis of Reports on Controlled Clinical Trials.* Geneva: World Health Organization.

134. Zhao, Z.-Q. (2008) 'Neural mechanism underlying acupuncture analgesia.' *Progress in Neurobiology 85*, 4, 355–375.

135. Lee, M.S. and Ernst, E. (2011) 'Acupuncture for pain: An overview of Cochrane reviews.' *Chinese Journal of Integrative Medicine 17*, 3, 187–189.

136. Dodin, S., Blanchet, C., Marc, I. *et al.* (2013) 'Acupuncture for menopausal hot flushes.' *Cochrane Database of Systematic Reviews.* Available at www.ncbi.nlm.nih.gov/pubmed/23897589, accessed on 29 February 2016.

137. Chiu, H.-Y., Pan, C.-H., Shyu, Y.-K., Han, B.-C. and Tsai, P.-S. (2015) 'Effects of acupuncture on menopause-related symptoms and quality of life in women on natural menopause: A meta-analysis of randomized controlled trials.' *Menopause 22*, 2, 1.

138. Blunt, E. (2006) 'Foot reflexology.' *Holistic Nursing Practice 20*, 5, 257–259.

139. Ernst, E. and Köder, K. (1997) 'An overview of reflexology.' *European Journal of General Practice 3*, 2, 52–57.

140. Ernst, E. and Köder, K. (1997) 'An overview of reflexology.' *European Journal of General Practice 3*, 2, 52–57.

141. Tiran, D. and Chummun, H. (2005) 'The physiological basis of reflexology and its use as a potential diagnostic tool.' *Complementary Therapies in Clinical Practice 11*, 1, 58–64.

142. McCullough, J.E.M., Liddle, S.D., Sinclair, M., Close, C. and Hughes, C.M. (2014) 'The physiological and biochemical outcomes associated with a reflexology treatment: A systematic review.' *Evidence-Based Complementary and Alternative Medicine.* doi:10.1155/2014/502123.

143. Williamson, J., White, A., Hart, A. and Ernst, E. (2002) 'Randomised controlled trial of reflexology for menopausal symptoms.' *BJOG: An International Journal of Obstetrics & Gynaecology 109*, 9, 1050–1055.

144. Ernst, E., Posadzki, P. and Lee, M.S. (2011) 'Reflexology: An update of a systematic review of randomised clinical trials.' *Maturitas 68*, 2, 116–120.

145. Asltoghiri, M. and Ghodsi, Z. (2012) 'The effects of reflexology on sleep disorder in menopausal women.' *Procedia-Social and Behavioral Sciences 31*, 242–246.

146. Williamson, J., White, A., Hart, A. and Ernst, E. (2002) 'Randomised controlled trial of reflexology for menopausal symptoms.' *BJOG: An International Journal of Obstetrics & Gynaecology 109*, 9, 1050–1055.

147. Bornhöft, G. and Matthiessen, P. (2011) *Homeopathy in Healthcare: Effectiveness, Appropriateness, Safety, Costs.* Berlin, Heidelberg: Springer Science & Business Media.

148. House of Commons (2009–10) Science and Technology Committee. Fourth Report. Evidence Check 2: Homeopathy. Available at www.publications. parliament.uk/pa/cm200910/cmselect/cmsctech/45/45.pdf, accessed on 31 March 2016.

149. Barnes, P.M., Bloom, B. and Nahin R.L. (2008) *Complementary and Alternative Medicine Use Among Adults and Children: United States, 2007.* National Health Statistics Reports; no 12. Hyattsville, MD: National Center for Health Statistics. Available at www.cdc.gov/nchs/data/nhsr/nhsr012.pdf, accessed on 31 March 2016.

150. Griffith, C. (2005) *The Companion to Homeopathy: The Practitioner's Guide.* New York, NY: Sterling Publishing Company, Inc.

151. Relton, C. and Weatherley-Jones, E. (2005) 'Homeopathy service in a National Health Service community menopause clinic: Audit of clinical outcomes.' *British Menopause Society Journal 11*, 2, 72–73.

152. Thompson, E.A. and Relton, C. (2009) 'Designing clinical trials of homeopathy for menopausal symptoms: A review of the literature.' *Menopause International 15*, 1, 31–34.

153. Jahnke, R., Larkey, L., Rogers, C., Etnier, J. and Lin, F. (2010) 'A comprehensive review of health benefits of Qigong and Tai Chi.' *American Journal of Health Promotion 24*, 6, e1–e25.

154. Jahnke, R., Larkey, L., Rogers, C., Etnier, J. and Lin, F. (2010) 'A comprehensive review of health benefits of Qigong and Tai Chi.' *American Journal of Health Promotion 24*, 6, e1–e25.

155. Chan, K., Qin, L., Lau, M. *et al.* (2004) 'A randomized, prospective study of the effects of Tai Chi Chun exercise on bone mineral density in postmenopausal women.' *Archives of Physical Medicine and Rehabilitation 85*, 5, 717–722.

156. Wayne, P.M., Kiel, D.P., Krebs, D.E. *et al.* (2007) 'The effects of Tai Chi on bone mineral density in postmenopausal women: A systematic review.' *Archives of Physical Medicine and Rehabilitation 88*, 5, 673–680.

157. Peng, W., Adams, J., Hickman, L. and Sibbritt, D.W. (2016) 'Longitudinal analysis of associations between women's consultations with complementary and alternative medicine practitioners/use of self-prescribed complementary and alternative medicine and menopause-related symptoms, 2007–2010.' *Menopause 23*, 1, 74–80.

158. Woods, N.F., Mitchell, E.S., Schnall, J.G. *et al.* (2014) 'Effects of mind-body therapies on symptom clusters during the menopausal transition.' *Climacteric 17*, 1, 10–22.

159. Hirschberg, A.L. (2012) 'Sex hormones, appetite and eating behaviour in women.' *Maturitas 71*, 3, 248–256.

160. Fowler, S.P., Williams, K., Resendez, R.G., Hunt, K.J., Hazuda, H.P. and Stern, M.P. (2008) 'Fueling the obesity epidemic? Artificially sweetened beverage use and long-term weight gain.' *Obesity 16*, 8, 1894–1900.

161. Green, E. and Murphy, C. (2012) 'Altered processing of sweet taste in the brain of diet soda drinkers.' *Physiology and Behavior 107*, 4, 560–567.

162. Mason, A.E., Daubenmier, J., Moran, P.J. *et al.* (2014) 'Increases in mindful eating predict reductions in consumption of sweets and desserts: Data from the Supporting Health by Integrating Nutrition and Exercise (SHINE) clinical trial.' *The Journal of Alternative and Complementary Medicine 20*, 5, A17–A17.

163. Beshara, M., Hutchinson, A.D. and Wilson, C. (2013) 'Does mindfulness matter? Everyday mindfulness, mindful eating and self-reported serving size of energy dense foods among a sample of South Australian adults.' *Appetite 67*, 25–29.

164. Timlin, M.T. and Pereira, M.A. (2007) 'Breakfast frequency and quality in the etiology of adult obesity and chronic diseases.' *Nutrition Reviews 65*, 6, 268.

165. Farshchi, H.R., Taylor, M.A. and Macdonald, I.A. (2005) 'Deleterious effects of omitting breakfast on insulin sensitivity and fasting lipid profiles in healthy lean women.' *The American Journal of Clinical Nutrition 81*, 2, 388–396.

166. Howe, T.E., Shea, B., Dawson, L.J. *et al.* (2011) 'Exercise for preventing and treating osteoporosis in postmenopausal women'. *Cochrane Database of Systematic Reviews 7.* doi: 10.1002/14651858.CD000333.pub2.

167. Manson, J.E., Greenland, P., LaCroix, A.Z. *et al.* (2002) 'Walking compared with vigorous exercise for the prevention of cardiovascular events in women.' *New England Journal of Medicine 347*, 10, 716–725.

168. Manson, J.E., Greenland, P., LaCroix, A.Z. *et al.* (2002) 'Walking compared with vigorous exercise for the prevention of cardiovascular events in women.' *New England Journal of Medicine 347*, 10, 716–725.

169. Carpenter, C.L., Ross, R.K., Paganini-Hill, A. and Bernstein, L. (2003) 'Effect of family history, obesity and exercise on breast cancer risk among postmenopausal women.' *International Journal of Cancer 106*, 1, 96–102.

170. Foley, D., Ancoli-Israel, S., Britz, P. and Walsh, J. (2004) 'Sleep disturbances and chronic disease in older adults: Results of the 2003 National Sleep Foundation Sleep in America Survey.' *Journal of Psychosomatic Research 56*, 5, 497–502.

171. Hysing, M., Pallesen, S., Stormark, K.M., Jakobsen, R., Lundervold, A.J. and Sivertsen, B. (2015) 'Sleep and use of electronic devices in adolescence: Results from a large population-based study.' *BMJ Open 5*, 1, e006748.

172. Exelmans, L. and Van den Bulck, J. (2015) 'Sleep quality is negatively related to video gaming volume in adults.' *Journal of Sleep Research 24*, 2, 189–196.

173. Chang, A.-M., Aeschbach, D., Duffy, J.F. and Czeisler, C.A. (2015) 'Evening use of light-emitting eReaders negatively affects sleep, circadian timing, and next-morning alertness.' *Proceedings of the National Academy of Sciences 112*, 4, 1232–1237.

174. Ebrahim, I.O., Shapiro, C.M., Williams, A.J. and Fenwick, P.B. (2013) 'Alcohol and sleep I: Effects on normal sleep.' *Alcoholism: Clinical and Experimental Research 37*, 4, 539–549.

175. Pilcher, J.J., Michalowski, K.R. and Carrigan, R.D. (2001) 'The prevalence of daytime napping and its relationship to nighttime sleep.' *Behavioral Medicine 27*, 2, 71–76.

176. Polo-Kantola, P. and Erkkola, R. (2004) 'Sleep and the menopause.' *British Menopause Society Journal 10*, 4, 145–150.

177. Montplaisir, J., Lorrain, J., Denesle, R. and Petit, D. (2001) 'Sleep in menopause: Differential effects of two forms of hormone replacement therapy.' *Menopause 8*, 1, 10–16.

178. Freedman, R.R. and Roehrs, T.A. (2007) 'Sleep disturbance in menopause.' *Menopause 14*, 5, 826–829.

179. Hsu, H.-C. and Lin, M.-H. (2005) 'Exploring quality of sleep and its related factors among menopausal women.' *Journal of Nursing Research 13*, 2, 153–164.

180. Dennerstein, L., Lehert, P. and Burger, H. (2005) 'The relative effects of hormones and relationship factors on sexual function of women through the natural menopausal transition.' *Fertility and Sterility 84*, 1, 174–180.

181. Cohen, S., Gottlieb, B.H. and Underwood, L.G. (2000) 'Social relationships and health.' In S. Cohen, L. Underwood, and B. Gottlieb (eds) *Measuring and Intervening in Social Support.* New York: Oxford University Press.

182. Uchino, B.N. (2006) 'Social support and health: A review of physiological processes potentially underlying links to disease outcomes.' *Journal of Behavioral Medicine 29*, 4, 377–387.

183. Mikal, J.P., Rice, R.E., Abeyta, A. and DeVilbiss, J. (2013) 'Transition, stress and computer-mediated social support.' *Computers in Human Behavior 29*, 5, A40–A53.

184. Barak, A., Boniel-Nissim, M. and Suler, J. (2008) 'Fostering empowerment in online support groups.' *Computers in Human Behavior 24*, 5, 1867–1883.

185. National Collaborating Centre for Women and Children's Health (2015) *Menopause: Diagnosis and Management.* NICE guidelines [NG23]. Available at www.nice.org.uk/guidance/ng23/ifp/chapter/about-this-information, accessed on 12 January 2016.

186. de Villiers, T.J., Gass, M.L., Haines, C.J. *et al.* (2013) 'Global consensus statement on menopausal hormone therapy.' *Climacteric 16*, 2, 203–204.

187. Canonico, M., Oger, E., Plu-Bureau, G. *et al.* (2007) 'Hormone therapy and venous thromboembolism among postmenopausal women: Impact of the route of estrogen administration and progestogens: The ESTHER study.' *Circulation 115*, 7, 840–845.

188. Whelan, A.M., Jurgens, T.M. and Trinacty, M. (2011) 'Defining bioidentical hormones for menopause-related symptoms.' *Pharm Pract (Granada) 9*, 1, 16–22.

189. Løkkegaard, E., Andreasen, A.H., Jacobsen, R.K., Nielsen, L.H., Agger, C. and Lidegaard, Ø. (2008) 'Hormone therapy and risk of myocardial infarction: A national register study.' *European Heart Journal 29*, 21, 2660–2668.

190. Sitruk-Ware, R., Bricaire, C., De Lignieres, B., Yaneva, H. and Mauvais-Jarvis, P. (1987) 'Oral micronized progesterone. Bioavailability pharmacokinetics, pharmacological and therapeutic implications--a review.' *Contraception 36*, 4, 373–402.

191. Wilson, R.A. (1966) *Feminine Forever.* London: W.H. Allen.

192. Reuben, D.R. (1970) *Everything You Always Wanted to Know About Sex (But Were Afraid to Ask).* W. H. Allen/Virgin Books.

193. Smith, D.C., Prentice, R., Thompson, D.J. and Herrmann, W.L. (1975) 'Association of exogenous estrogen and endometrial carcinoma.' *New England Journal of Medicine 293*, 23, 1164–7.

194. Ziel, H.K., Finkle, W.D. (1975) 'Increased risk of endometrial carcinoma among users of conjugated estrogens.' *New England Journal of Medicine 293*, 23, 1167–1170.

195. Gambrell, R.D. Jr, Massey, F.M., Castaneda,T.A., Ugenas, A.J., Ricci, C.A. and Wright, J.M. (1980) 'Use of the progestogen challenge test to reduce the risk of endometrial cancer.' *Obstetrics and Gynecology 55*, 6, 732–8.

196. de Villiers, T.J., Gass, M.L., Haines, C.J. *et al.* (2013) 'Global consensus statement on menopausal hormone therapy.' *Climacteric 16*, 2, 203–204.

197. Panay, N., Hamoda, H., Arya, R. and Savvas, M. (2013) 'The 2013 British Menopause Society & Women's Health Concern recommendations on hormone replacement therapy.' *Menopause International 19*, 2, 59–68.

198. Panay, N. (2004) 'Hormone replacement therapy: The way forward.' *Journal of Family Planning and Reproductive Health Care 30*, 1, 21–24.

199. Panay, N., Hamoda, H., Arya, R. and Savvas, M. (2013) 'The 2013 British Menopause Society & Women's Health Concern recommendations on hormone replacement therapy.' *Menopause International 19*, 2, 59–68.

200. Cody, J.D., Richardson, K., Moehrer, B., Hextall, A., Glazener, C.M. (2009) 'Oestrogen therapy for urinary incontinence in post-menopausal women.' *Cochrane Database of Systematic Reviews 4*. doi: 10.1002/14651858.CD001405.pub2.

201. Simon, J.A. and Maamari, R.V. (2013) 'Ultra-low-dose vaginal estrogen tablets for the treatment of postmenopausal vaginal atrophy.' *Climacteric 16* Suppl 1, 37–43.

202. Hendrix, S.L., Cochrane, B.B., Nygaard, I.E. et al. (2005) 'Effects of estrogen with and without progestin on urinary incontinence.' *Journal of the American Medical Association 23*, 293(8), 935–948.

203. National Collaborating Centre for Women and Children's Health (2015) *Menopause: Diagnosis and Management.* NICE guidelines [NG23]. Available at www.nice.org.uk/guidance/ng23/evidence/full-guideline-559549261, accessed on 29 February 2016.

204. Schmidt, P. (2012) 'The 2012 hormone therapy position statement of The North American Menopause Society.' *Menopause 19*, 3, 257–271.

205. Panay, N., Hamoda, H., Arya, R. and Savvas, M. (2013) 'The 2013 British Menopause Society & Women's Health Concern recommendations on hormone replacement therapy.' *Menopause International 19*, 2, 59–68.

206. Schmidt, P. (2012) 'The 2012 hormone therapy position statement of The North American Menopause Society.' *Menopause 19*, 3, 257–271.

207. de Villiers, T.J., Gass, M.L., Haines, C.J. *et al.* (2013) 'Global consensus statement on menopausal hormone therapy.' *Climacteric 16*, 2, 203–204.

208. Panay, N. (2004) 'Hormone replacement therapy: The way forward.' *Journal of Family Planning and Reproductive Health Care 30*, 1, 21–24.

209. Panay, N., Hamoda, H., Arya, R. and Savvas, M. (2013) 'The 2013 British Menopause Society & Women's Health Concern recommendations on hormone replacement therapy.' *Menopause International 19*, 2, 59–68.

210. Harman, S.M., Black, D.M., Naftolin, F. *et al.* (2014) 'Arterial imaging outcomes and cardiovascular risk factors in recently menopausal women: A randomized trial.' *Annals of Internal Medicine 161*, 4, 249–260.

211. L'hermite, M., Simoncini, T., Fuller, S. and Genazzani, A.R. (2008) 'Could transdermal estradiol + progesterone be a safer postmenopausal HRT? A review.' *Maturitas 60*, 3–4, 185–201.

212. Boardman, H.M., Hartley, L., Eisinga, A. *et al.* (2015) 'Hormone therapy for preventing cardiovascular disease in post-menopausal women.' *Cochrane Database of Systematic Review 3*, CD002229.

213. Schmidt, P. (2012) 'The 2012 hormone therapy position statement of The North American Menopause Society.' *Menopause 19*, 3, 257–271.

214. de Villiers, T.J., Gass, M.L., Haines, C.J. *et al.* (2013) 'Global consensus statement on menopausal hormone therapy.' *Climacteric 16*, 2, 203–204.

215. Rossouw, J.E., Anderson, G.L., Prentice, R.L. *et al.* (2002) 'Risks and benefits of estrogen plus progestin in healthy postmenopausal women: Principal results from the Women's Health Initiative randomized controlled trial.' *Journal of the American Medical Association 288*, 3, 321–333.

216. Schmidt, P. (2012) 'The 2012 hormone therapy position statement of The North American Menopause Society.' *Menopause 19*, 3, 257–271.

217. Jeng, M.H., Parker, C.J. and Jordan, V.C. (1992) 'Estrogenic potential of progestins in oral contraceptives to stimulate human breast cancer cell proliferation.' *Cancer Research 52*, 23, 6539–6546.

218. Catherino, W.H., Jeng, M.H. and Jordan, V.C. (1993) 'Norgestrel and gestodene stimulate breast cancer cell growth through an oestrogen receptor mediated mechanism.' *British Journal of Cancer 67*, 5, 945–952.

219. Collaborative Group on Hormonal Factors in Breast Cancer (1997) 'Breast cancer and hormone replacement therapy: Collaborative reanalysis of data from 51 epidemiological studies of 52,705 women with breast cancer and 108,411 women without breast cancer. Collaborative group on hormonal factors in breast cancer.' *Lancet 350*, 9084, 1047–1059.

220. Beral, V., and Million Women Study Collaborators (2003) 'Breast cancer and hormone-replacement therapy in the Million Women Study.' *Lancet 362*, 9382, 419–427.

221. National Collaborating Centre for Women and Children's Health (2015) *Menopause: Diagnosis and Management.* NICE guidelines [NG23]. Available at www.nice.org.uk/guidance/ng23/evidence/full-guideline-559549261, accessed on 29 February 2016.

222. Rossouw, J.E., Anderson, G.L., Prentice, R.L. *et al.* (2002) 'Risks and benefits of estrogen plus progestin in healthy postmenopausal women: Principal results from the Women's Health Initiative randomized controlled trial.' *Journal of the American Medical Association 288*, 3, 321–333.

223. Manson, J.E., Chlebowski, R.T., Stefanick, M.L. et al. (2013) 'Menopausal hormone therapy and health outcomes during the intervention and extended poststopping phases of the Women's Health Initiative randomized trials.' *Journal of the American Medical Association 310*, 13, 1353–1368.

224. L'hermite, M., Simoncini, T., Fuller, S. and Genazzani, A.R. (2008) 'Could transdermal estradiol + progesterone be a safer postmenopausal HRT? A review.' *Maturitas 60*, 3–4, 185–201.

225. Panay, N. (2004) 'Hormone replacement therapy: The way forward.' *Journal of Family Planning and Reproductive Health Care 30*, 1, 21–24.

226. Shapiro, S., de Villiers, T.J., Pines, A. *et al.* (2014) 'Risks and benefits of hormone therapy: Has medical dogma now been overturned?' *Climacteric 17*, 3, 215–222.

227. Ewertz, M., Mellemkjaer, L., Poulsen, A.H. *et al.* (2005) 'Hormone use for menopausal symptoms and risk of breast cancer. A Danish cohort study.' *British Journal of Cancer 92*, 7, 1293–1297.

228. Anderson, G.L., Limacher, M., Assaf, A.R. *et al.* (2004) 'Effects of conjugated equine estrogen in postmenopausal women with hysterectomy: The Women's Health Initiative randomized controlled trial.' *Journal of the American Medical Association 291*, 14, 1701–1712.

229. L'hermite, M., Simoncini, T., Fuller, S. and Genazzani, A.R. (2008) 'Could transdermal estradiol + progesterone be a safer postmenopausal HRT? A review.' *Maturitas 60*, 3–4, 185–201.

230. Stahlberg, C., Pedersen, A.T., Lynge, E. *et al.* (2004) 'Increased risk of breast cancer following different regimens of hormone replacement therapy frequently used in Europe.' *International Journal of Cancer 109*, 5, 721–727.

231. Fitzpatrick, L.A. and Good, A. (1999) 'Micronized progesterone: Clinical indications and comparison with current treatments.' *Fertility and Sterility 72*, 3, 389–397.

232. Gompel, A. (2012) 'Micronized progesterone and its impact on the endometrium and breast vs. progestogens.' *Climacteric 15*, Suppl 1, 18–25.

233. Wood, C.E., Register, T.C., Lees, C.J., Chen, H., Kimrey, S. and Cline, J.M. (2007) 'Effects of estradiol with micronized progesterone or medroxyprogesterone acetate on risk markers for breast cancer in postmenopausal monkeys.' *Breast Cancer Research and Treatment 101*, 2, 125–134.

234. de Villiers, T.J., Gass, M.L., Haines, C.J. *et al.* (2013) 'Global consensus statement on menopausal hormone therapy.' *Climacteric 16*, 2, 203–204.

235. Schierbeck, L.L., Rejnmark, L., Tofteng, C.L., *et al.* (2012) 'Effect of hormone replacement therapy on cardiovascular events in recently postmenopausal women: randomised trial.' *British Medical Journal 345*:e6409.

236. Hodis, H.N., Mack, W.J., Shoupe, D. et al. (2014) 'Testing the menopausal hormone therapy timing hypothesis: The Early Vs Late Intervention Trial with Estradiol.' *Circulation 130*: A13283.

237. L'hermite, M., Simoncini, T., Fuller, S. and Genazzani, A.R. (2008) 'Could transdermal estradiol + progesterone be a safer postmenopausal HRT? A review.' *Maturitas 60*, 3–4, 185–201.

238. L'hermite, M., Simoncini, T., Fuller, S. and Genazzani, A.R. (2008) 'Could transdermal estradiol + progesterone be a safer postmenopausal HRT? A review.' *Maturitas 60*, 3–4, 185–201.

239. Boardman, H.M., Hartley, L., Eisinga, A. *et al.* (2015) 'Hormone therapy for preventing cardiovascular disease in post-menopausal women.' *Cochrane Database of Systematic Review 3*, CD002229.

240. Panay, N., Hamoda, H., Arya, R. and Savvas, M. (2013) 'The 2013 British Menopause Society & Women's Health Concern recommendations on hormone replacement therapy.' *Menopause International 19*, 2, 59–68.

241. Canonico, M., Oger, E., Plu-Bureau, G. *et al.* (2007) 'Hormone therapy and venous thromboembolism among postmenopausal women: Impact of the route of estrogen administration and progestogens: The ESTHER study.' *Circulation 115*, 7, 840–845.

242. Panay, N., Hamoda, H., Arya, R. and Savvas, M. (2013) 'The 2013 British Menopause Society & Women's Health Concern recommendations on hormone replacement therapy.' *Menopause International 19*, 2, 59–68.

243. Schmidt, P. (2012) 'The 2012 hormone therapy position statement of The North American Menopause Society.' *Menopause 19*, 3, 257–271.

244. Panay, N. (2005) The menopause and HRT: Where are we now?' *The New Generalist 3*, 4, 16–19.

245. Panay, N., Hamoda, H., Arya, R. and Savvas, M. (2013) 'The 2013 British Menopause Society & Women's Health Concern recommendations on hormone replacement therapy.' *Menopause International 19*, 2, 59–68.

246. Rossouw, J.E., Anderson, G.L., Prentice, R.L. *et al.* (2002) 'Risks and benefits of estrogen plus progestin in healthy postmenopausal women: Principal results from the Women's Health Initiative randomized controlled trial.' *Journal of the American Medical Association 288*, 3, 321–333.

247. Rossouw, J.E., Prentice, R.L., Manson, J.E. *et al.* (2007) 'Postmenopausal hormone therapy and risk of cardiovascular disease by age and years since menopause.' *Journal of the American Medical Association 297*, 13, 1465–1477.

248. de Villiers, T.J., Gass, M.L., Haines, C.J. *et al.* (2013) 'Global consensus statement on menopausal hormone therapy.' *Climacteric 16*, 2, 203–204.

249. Liu, B., Beral, V., Balkwill, A. *et al.* (2008) 'Gallbladder disease and use of transdermal versus oral hormone replacement therapy in postmenopausal women: Prospective cohort study.' *British Medical Journal 337*, a386.

250. Liu, B., Beral, V., Balkwill, A. *et al.* (2008) 'Gallbladder disease and use of transdermal versus oral hormone replacement therapy in postmenopausal women: Prospective cohort study.' *British Medical Journal 337*, a386.

251. Schmidt, P. (2012) 'The 2012 hormone therapy position statement of The North American Menopause Society.' *Menopause 19*, 3, 257–271.

252. Panay, N., Hamoda, H., Arya, R. and Savvas, M. (2013) 'The 2013 British Menopause Society & Women's Health Concern recommendations on hormone replacement therapy.' *Menopause International 19*, 2, 59–68.

253. Beral, V., Bull, D., Green, J., Reeves, G. and Million Women Study Collaborators (2007) 'Ovarian cancer and hormone replacement therapy in the Million Women Study.' *Lancet 369*, 9574, 1703–1710.

254. Collaborative Group on Epidemiological Studies of Ovarian Cancer, Beral, V., Gaitskell, K., Hermon, C., Moser, K., Reeves, G. and Peto, R. (2015) 'Menopausal hormone use and ovarian cancer risk: Individual participant meta-analysis of 52 epidemiological studies.' *Lancet 385*, 9980, 1835–1842.

255. Panay, N., Hamoda, H., Arya, R. and Savvas, M. (2013) 'The 2013 British Menopause Society & Women's Health Concern recommendations on hormone replacement therapy.' *Menopause International 19*, 2, 59–68.

256. Panay, N. (2005) The menopause and HRT: Where are we now?' *The New Generalist 3*, 4, 16–19.

257. Chlebowski, R.T., Schwartz, A.G., Wakelee, H. *et al.* (2009) 'Oestrogen plus progestin and lung cancer in postmenopausal women (Women's Health Initiative trial): A post-hoc analysis of a randomised controlled trial.' *Lancet 374*, 9697, 1243–1251.

258. Panay, N., Hamoda, H., Arya, R. and Savvas, M. (2013) 'The 2013 British Menopause Society & Women's Health Concern recommendations on hormone replacement therapy.' *Menopause International 19*, 2, 59–68.

259. Greendale, G.A., Huang, M.H., Wight, R.G. *et al.* (2009) 'Effects of the menopause transition and hormone use on cognitive performance in midlife women.' *Neurology 72*, 21, 1850–1857.

260. Marjoribanks, J., Farquhar, C., Roberts, H. and Lethaby, A. (2012) 'Long term hormone therapy for perimenopausal and postmenopausal women.' *Cochrane Database of Systematic Review 7*, CD004143.

261. Panay, N. (2004) 'Hormone replacement therapy: The way forward.' *Journal of Family Planning and Reproductive Health Care 30*, 1, 21–24.

262. Salpeter, S.R., Walsh, J.M., Greyber, E., Ormiston, T.M. and Salpeter, E.E. (2004) 'Mortality associated with hormone replacement therapy in younger and older women: A meta-analysis.' *Journal of General Internal Medicine 19*, 7, 791–804.

263. Schmidt, P. (2012) 'The 2012 hormone therapy position statement of The North American Menopause Society.' *Menopause 19*, 3, 257–271.

264. Simon, J.A. (2012) 'What's new in hormone replacement therapy: Focus on transdermal estradiol and micronized progesterone.' *Climacteric 15*, Suppl 1, 3–10.

265. L'hermite, M., Simoncini, T., Fuller, S. and Genazzani, A.R. (2008) 'Could transdermal estradiol + progesterone be a safer postmenopausal HRT? A review.' *Maturitas 60*, 3–4, 185–201.

266. de Villiers, T.J., Gass, M.L., Haines, C.J. *et al.* (2013) 'Global consensus statement on menopausal hormone therapy.' *Climacteric 16*, 2, 203–204.

267. Schmidt, P. (2012) 'The 2012 hormone therapy position statement of The North American Menopause Society.' *Menopause 19*, 3, 257–271.

268. Panay, N., Hamoda, H., Arya, R. and Savvas, M. (2013) 'The 2013 British Menopause Society & Women's Health Concern recommendations on hormone replacement therapy.' *Menopause International 19*, 2, 59–68.

269. Schmidt, P. (2012) 'The 2012 hormone therapy position statement of The North American Menopause Society.' *Menopause 19*, 3, 257–271.

270. Panay, N., Hamoda, H., Arya, R. and Savvas, M. (2013) 'The 2013 British Menopause Society & Women's Health Concern recommendations on hormone replacement therapy.' *Menopause International 19*, 2, 59–68.

271. Lethaby, A., Hussain, M., Rishworth, J.R. and Rees, M.C. (2015) 'Progesterone or progestogen-releasing intrauterine systems for heavy menstrual bleeding.' *Cochrane Database of Systematic Review 4*, CD002126.

272. Panay, N., Hamoda, H., Arya, R. and Savvas, M. (2013) 'The 2013 British Menopause Society & Women's Health Concern recommendations on hormone replacement therapy.' *Menopause International 19*, 2, 59–68.

273. Panjari, M. and Davis, S.R. (2011) 'Vaginal DHEA to treat menopause related atrophy: A review of the evidence.' *Maturitas 70*, 1, 22–25.

274. Maclaran, K. and Panay, N. (2011) 'Managing low sexual desire in women.' *Women's Health (London England) 7*, 5, 571–581.

275. Zhang, F., Swanson, S.M., van Breemen, R.B. *et al.* (2001) 'Equine estrogen metabolite 4-hydroxyequilenin induces DNA damage in the rat mammary tissues: Formation of single-strand breaks, apurinic sites, stable adducts, and oxidized bases.' *Chemical Research in Toxicology 14*, 12, 1654–1659.

276. Lippert, T.H., Mueck, A.O. and Seeger, H. (2000) 'Is the use of conjugated equine oestrogens in hormone replacement therapy still appropriate?' *British Journal of Clinical Pharmacology 49*, 5, 489–490.

277. Panay, N., Hamoda, H., Arya, R. and Savvas, M. (2013) 'The 2013 British Menopause Society & Women's Health Concern recommendations on hormone replacement therapy.' *Menopause International 19*, 2, 59–68.

278. de Lignières, B. (1999) 'Oral micronized progesterone.' *Clinical Therapeutics 21*, 1, 41–60; discussion 41–42.

279. Fitzpatrick, L.A., Pace, C. and Wiita, B. (2000) 'Comparison of regimens containing oral micronized progesterone or medroxyprogesterone acetate on quality of life in postmenopausal women: A cross-sectional survey.' *Journal of Women's Health and Gender Based Medicine 9*, 4, 381–387.

280. Montplaisir, J., Lorrain, J., Denesle, R. and Petit, D. (2001) 'Sleep in menopause: differential effects of two forms of hormone replacement therapy.' *Menopause 8*, 1, 10–16.

281. Hargrove, J.T., Maxson, W.S., Wentz, A.C. and Burnett LS. (1989) 'Menopausal hormone replacement therapy with continuous daily oral micronized estradiol and progesterone.' *Obstetrics and Gynecology 73*, 4, 606–612.

282. Panay, N., Hamoda, H., Arya, R. and Savvas, M. (2013) 'The 2013 British Menopause Society & Women's Health Concern recommendations on hormone replacement therapy.' *Menopause International 19*, 2, 59–68.

283. Files, J.A., Ko, M.G. and Pruthi, S. (2011) 'Bioidentical hormone therapy.' *Mayo Clinic Proceedings 86*, 7, 673–680.

284. Files, J.A., Ko, M.G. and Pruthi, S. (2011) 'Bioidentical hormone therapy.' *Mayo Clinic Proceedings 86*, 7, 673–680.

285. Zhu, B.T., Han, G.Z., Shim, J.Y., Wen, Y. and Jiang, X.R. (2006) 'Quantitative structure-activity relationship of various endogenous estrogen metabolites for human estrogen receptor alpha and beta subtypes: Insights into the structural determinants favoring a differential subtype binding.' *Endocrinology 147*, 9, 4132–4150.

286. de Villiers, T.J., Gass, M.L., Haines, C.J. *et al.* (2013) 'Global consensus statement on menopausal hormone therapy.' *Climacteric 16*, 2, 203–204.

287. Cummings, S.R., Ettinger, B., Delmas, P.D. *et al.* (2008) 'The effects of tibolone in older postmenopausal women.' *New England Journal of Medicine 359*, 7, 697–708.

288. Nelson, H.D., Fu, R., Griffin, J.C., Nygren, P., Smith, M.E. and Humphrey, L. (2009) 'Systematic review: Comparative effectiveness of medications to reduce risk for primary breast cancer.' *Annals of Internal Medicine 151*, 10, 703–715, W-226–735.

289. UK Government (2007) 'MHRA. Drug Safety Update, Tibolone: Benefit-risk balance.' Available at www.gov.uk/drug-safety-update/tibolone-benefit-risk-balance#fn:2, accessed on 05 August 2015.

290. Bundred, N.J., Kenemans, P., Yip, C.H. *et al.* (2012) 'Tibolone increases bone mineral density but also relapse in breast cancer survivors: LIBERATE trial bone substudy.' *Breast Cancer Research 14*, 1, R13.

291. Nelson, H.D., Fu, R., Griffin, J.C., Nygren, P., Smith, M.E. and Humphrey L. (2009) 'Systematic review: Comparative effectiveness of medications to reduce risk for primary breast cancer.' *Annals of Internal Medicine 151*, 10, 703–715, W-226–735.

292. Cummings, S.R., Ettinger, B., Delmas, P.D., *et al.* (2008) 'The effects of tibolone in older postmenopausal women.' *New England Journal of Medicine 359*, 7, 697–708.

293. Cummings, S.R., Ettinger, B., Delmas, P.D., *et al.* (2008) 'The effects of tibolone in older postmenopausal women.' *New England Journal of Medicine 359*, 7, 697–708.

294. Beral, V., and Million Women Study Collaborators (2003) 'Breast cancer and hormone-replacement therapy in the Million Women Study.' *Lancet 362*, 9382, 419–427.

295. Stahlberg, C., Pedersen, A.T., Lynge, E. *et al.* (2004) 'Increased risk of breast cancer following different regimens of hormone replacement therapy frequently used in Europe.' *International Journal of Cancer 109*, 5, 721–727.

296. Cummings, S.R., Ettinger, B., Delmas, P.D. *et al.* (2008) 'The effects of tibolone in older postmenopausal women.' *New England Journal of Medicine 359*, 7, 697–708.

297. Nelson, H.D., Fu, R., Griffin, J.C., Nygren, P., Smith, M.E. and Humphrey L. (2009) 'Systematic review: Comparative effectiveness of medications to reduce risk for primary breast cancer.' *Annals of Internal Medicine 151*, 10, 703–715, W-226–735.

298. Nelson, H.D., Fu, R., Griffin, J.C., Nygren, P., Smith, M.E. and Humphrey L. (2009) 'Systematic review: Comparative effectiveness of medications to reduce risk for primary breast cancer.' *Annals of Internal Medicine 151*, 10, 703–715, W-226–735.

299. Nelson, H.D., Fu, R., Griffin, J.C., Nygren, P., Smith, M.E. and Humphrey L. (2009) 'Systematic review: Comparative effectiveness of medications to reduce risk for primary breast cancer.' *Annals of Internal Medicine 151*, 10, 703–715, W-226–735.

300. Vehmanen, L., Elomaa, I., Blomqvist, C. and Saarto, T. (2006) 'Tamoxifen treatment after adjuvant chemotherapy has opposite effects on bone mineral density in premenopausal patients depending on menstrual status.' *Journal of Clinical Oncology 24*, 4, 675–680.

301. Khadilkar, S. (2012) 'Hormone replacement therapy: an update. *Journal of Obstetrics and Gynaecology of India 62*, 3, 261–265.

302. Stearns, V., Beebe, K.L., Iyengar, M., Dube, E. (2003) 'Paroxetine controlled release in the treatment of menopausal hot flashes: A randomized controlled trial.' *Journal of the American Medical Association 289*, 21, 2827–2834.

303. Loprinzi, C.L., Sloan, J.A., Perez, E.A. *et al.* (2002) 'Phase III evaluation of fluoxetine for treatment of hot flashes.' *Journal of Clinical Oncology 20*, 6, 1578–1583.

304. Carpenter, J.S., Guthrie, K.A., Larson, J.C. *et al.* (2012) 'Effect of escitalopram on hot flash interference: A randomized, controlled trial.' *Fertility and Sterility 97*, 6, 1399–1404. e1.

305. Suvanto-Luukkonen, E., Koivunen, R., Sundström, H. *et al.* (2005) 'Citalopram and fluoxetine in the treatment of postmenopausal symptoms: A prospective, randomized, 9-month, placebo-controlled, double-blind study.' *Menopause 12*, 1, 18–26.

306. Shams, T., Firwana, B., Habib, F. *et al.* (2014) 'SSRIs for hot flashes: A systematic review and meta-analysis of randomized trials.' *Journal of General Internal Medicine 29*, 1, 204–213.

307. Loprinzi, C.L., Kugler, J.W., Sloan, J.A. *et al.* (2000) 'Venlafaxine in management of hot flashes in survivors of breast cancer: A randomised controlled trial.' *Lancet 356*, 9247, 2059–2063.

308. Panay, N., Hamoda, H., Arya, R. and Savvas, M. (2013) 'The 2013 British Menopause Society & Women's Health Concern recommendations on hormone replacement therapy.' *Menopause International 19*, 2, 59–68.

309. Jane, F.M. and Davis, S.R. (2014) 'A practitioner's toolkit for managing the menopause.' *Climacteric 17*, 5, 564–579.

310. Butt, D.A., Lock, M., Lewis, J.E., Ross, S. and Moineddin, R. (2008) 'Gabapentin for the treatment of menopausal hot flashes: A randomized controlled trial.' *Menopause 15*, 2, 310–318.

311. Toulis, K.A., Tzellos, T., Kouvelas, D. and Goulis, D.G. (2009) 'Gabapentin for the treatment of hot flashes in women with natural or tamoxifen-induced menopause: A systematic review and meta-analysis.' *Clinical Therapeutics 31*, 2, 221–235.

312. Panay, N., Hamoda, H., Arya, R. and Savvas, M. (2013) 'The 2013 British Menopause Society & Women's Health Concern recommendations on hormone replacement therapy.' *Menopause International 19*, 2, 59–68.

313. Panay, N., Hamoda, H., Arya, R. and Savvas, M. (2013) 'The 2013 British Menopause Society & Women's Health Concern recommendations on hormone replacement therapy.' *Menopause International 19*, 2, 59–68.

314. Rada, G., Capurro, D., Pantoja, T. *et al.* (2010) 'Non-hormonal interventions for hot flushes in women with a history of breast cancer.' *Cochrane Database of Systematic Review 9*, CD004923.

315. Jane, F.M. and Davis, S.R. (2014) 'A practitioner's toolkit for managing the menopause.' *Climacteric 17*, 5, 564–579.

316. North American Menopause Society (NAMS) (2015) 'Vaginal and Vulvar Comfort: Lubricants, Moisturisers, and Low-dose Vaginal Estrogen.' Available at www.menopause.org/for-women/sexual-health-menopause-online/effective-treatments-for-sexual-problems/vaginal-and-vulvar-comfort-lubricants-moisturizers-and-low-dose-vaginal-estrogen, accessed on 28 October 2015.

317. Khadilkar, S. (2012) 'Hormone replacement therapy: An update.' *Journal of Obstetircs and Gynaecology of India 62*, 3, 261-265.

318. Saita, Y., Ishijima, M. and Kaneko, K. (2015) 'Atypical femoral fractures and bisphosphonate use: Current evidence and clinical implications.' *Therapeutic Advances in Chronic Disease 6*, 4, 185–193.

319. Giusti, A., Hamdy, N.A., Dekkers, O.M., Ramautar, S.R., Dijkstra, S. and Papapoulos, S. (2011) 'Atypical fractures and bisphosphonate therapy: A cohort study of patients with femoral fracture with radiographic adjudication of fracture site and features.' *Bone 48*, 5, 966–971.

320. Lenart, B.A., Neviaser, A.S, Lyman, S. et al.(2009) 'Association of low-energy femoral fractures with prolonged bisphosphonate use: A case control study.' *Osteoporosis International 20*, 8, 1353–1362.

321. Park-Wyllie, L.Y., Mamdani, M.M., Juurlink, D.N. et al. (2011) 'Bisphosphonate use and the risk of subtrochanteric or femoral shaft fractures in older women.' *Journal of the American Medical Association 305*, 8, 783–789.

322. Schilcher, J., Michaëlsson, K. and Aspenberg, P. (2011) 'Bisphosphonate use and atypical fractures of the femoral shaft.' *New England Journal of Medicine 364*, 1, 1728–37.

323. Shane, E., Burr, D., Abrahamsen, B. *et al.* (2010) 'Atypical subtrochanteric and diaphyseal femoral fractures: Report of a task force of the American Society for Bone and Mineral Research.' *Journal of Bone and Mineral Research 25*, 11, 2267–294.

324. Food and Drug Administration (2011) Background document for meeting of Advisory Committee for Reproductive Health Drugs and Drug Safety and Risk Management Advisory Committee. September 9, 2011. Available at www.fda. gov/downloads/AdvisoryCommittees/CommitteesMeetingMaterials/Drugs/ DrugSafetyandRiskManagementAdvisoryCommittee/UCM270958.pdf, accessed on 14 January 2016.

325. Watts, N.B. and Diab, D.L. (2010) 'Long-term use of bisphosphonates in osteoporosis.' *Journal of Clinical Endocrinology and Metabolism 95*, 4, 1555–1565.

326. Järvinen, T.L., Michaëlsson, K., Jokihaara, J. *et al.* (2015) 'Overdiagnosis of bone fragility in the quest to prevent hip fracture.' *British Medical Journal 350*, h2088.

327. Gallacher, S.J. and Dixon, T. (2010) 'Impact of treatments for postmenopausal osteoporosis (bisphosphonates, parathyroid hormone, strontium ranelate, and denosumab) on bone quality: A systematic review.' *Calcified Tissue International 87*, 6, 469–484.

328. Nygård, O., Vollset, S.E., Refsum, H. *et al.* (1995) 'Total plasma homocysteine and cardiovascular risk profile: The Hordaland Homocysteine Study.' *Journal of the America Medical Association 274*, 19, 1526–1533.

329. Ciaccio, M. and Bellia, C. (2010) 'Hyperhomocysteinemia and cardiovascular risk: Effect of vitamin supplementation in risk reduction.' *Current Clinical Pharmacology 5*, 1, 30–36.

330. Martí-Carvajal, A.J., Solà, I., Lathyris, D., Karakitsiou, D.E. and Simancas-Racines, D. (2013) 'Homocysteine-lowering interventions for preventing cardiovascular events.' *Cochrane Database of Systematic Review 1*, CD006612.

331. Refsum, H., Nurk, E., Smith, A.D. *et al.* (2006) 'The Hordaland Homocysteine Study: A community-based study of homocysteine, its determinants, and associations with disease.' *Journal of Nutrition 136*, 6 Suppl, 1731S–1740S.

INDEX

Actonel 206
acupuncture 113–5
age
    average start of menopause 14
    HRT risk and 163–4
Ageless: The Naked Truth about
    Bioidentical Hormones 150
alcohol
    calculating units 61
    government guidelines 60
    risks associated with 61–2
    and sleep 137
Alora 188
alternative therapies see
    complementary and alternative
    medicine (CAM) therapies
Alzheimer's disease/dementia 32–4,
    86, 173–4
angelica (dong quai) 88
anovulatory cycles 21
antioxidants 58–9
anxiety 27, 78
attractiveness, sense of 45

bazedoxifene (BZA) 200–1
Beck, Aaron 92–3
beer 61
behavioural therapy see psychological/
    behavioural therapies
bioidentical hormone replacement
    therapy (BHRT)
    17beta-oestradiol 187–8, 190

breast cancer and 165–6
compounding pharmacies 189–92
oestrogen 187–8
overview of 148–50, 187
progesterone 188–9
pros and cons 192–3
safety of 167
testosterone 189
Wiley Protocol 149–50
Bisphenol A (BPA) 64, 67
bisphosphonates (BPs) 206–9, 211–2
black cohosh 83–5
blood clots 167–70
body image 41–3, 45
bone health see osteoporosis
breast cancer
    bioidentical hormones and 165–6
    breast screening 36–8
    checking your breasts 36
    HRT and 161–7
    overview of 34–5
    red clover and 78
    risk factors 35
    soya and risk for 74–5
    tamoxifen 75, 200
British Psychological Society 102–3

calcium 79–82
Chinese herbal medicine (CHM) 87–9
cholesterol 17 8
cider 61
Climara patch 187, 188

Clonidine 204–5
cognitive behavioural therapy (CBT)
92–6, 102–4
cognitive function, memory loss 32–4,
86, 173–4
colorectal cancer 159
comfort eating 132
complementary and alternative
medicine (CAM) therapies
acupuncture 113–5
Complementary and Natural
Healthcare Council (CNHC)
register 122
finding a reputable therapist 121–4
homeopathy 118–9
mind-body medicine 109
overview of 108–10
questions to ask prospective
therapist 122–4
reasons to use 110–1
reflexology 115–7
tai chi 119–20
telling your doctor about 124
yoga 111–3
Complementary and Natural
Healthcare Council (CNHC)
register 122
compounding pharmacies 189–92
confidence, increased 45–6
conjugated equine estrogens (CEE)
151, 154, 156, 185–6, 200–1
continuous combined regimen 181
contraceptive pill 161, 168, 182

decaffeinated drinks 137
deep vein thrombosis 167–70
dehydroepiandrosterone (DHEA)
184–5
dementia/Alzheimer's disease 32–4,
86, 173–4
depression 26–7, 78, 85–6, 139
diabetes, Type 2 38–40, 159
diary of symptoms 127–31
diet
comfort eating 132
decaffeinated drinks 137
diet drinks 132
energy density 54–6
'five a day' 58–9

fruit 58
Ketogenic 53
low-fat foods 132
Mediterranean style 60
omega oils 52
processed meat 50–1
red meat 50
salt 51
saturated fat 53
sugar 54
vegetables 58–9
dietary supplements
calcium 79–82
evening primrose oil 82–3
overview of 51, 69–70
phytoestrogens 71–9
red clover 77–8
soya 71–6
vitamin D 79–82
vitamin K 82
see also herbs
dong quai 88
drugs *see* bioidentical hormone
replacement therapy (BHRT);
Hormone Replacement Therapy
(HRT); medical management

early onset menopause 19–20, 181–2
Endocrine Disruption Exchange
(TEDX) 65
endocrine-disrupting chemicals
(EDCs) 20, 64–6
endometrial cancer 74–5, 173
energy density 54–6
environmental toxins 63–7
Esclim 188
essential fatty acids (EFAs) 52
Estrace 188
Estraderm 188
Estradiol 188
Estrasorb 188
evening primrose oil 82–3
Evorel 188
exercise
best types of 133–4
tai chi 119–20
walking 134–5
yoga 111–3

fats
    omega oils 52
    saturated fats 53
fight or flight response 91
filters, water 66
'five a day' 58–9
food *see* alcohol; diet; dietary
    supplements
food intolerances 62–3
Fosamax 206
freedom, increase in 46–7
fruit 58–9

Gabapentin 203–4
gallbladder disease 171
genetic factors 29
ginseng 86–7
glycemic index 56–8
glycemic load 56–8

Hatha yoga 113
headaches 24–6, 62, 156
Health and Care Professions Council
    (HCPC) 103–4
heart health
    cardiovascular disease (CVD) risk
        factors 31–2
    ginseng for 86
    HRT and 158–9, 167–71
    overview of advice 226–7
    palpitations 26
    red clover and 78
    soya and 75–6
herbs
    black cohosh 83–5
    Chinese herbal medicine (CHM)
        87–9
    dong quai 88
    ginseng 86–7
    St John's wort 85–6
    see also dietary supplements
hobbies 144
homeopathy 118–9
homocysteine 216–8
Hormone Replacement Therapy
    (HRT)
    age and risk 163–4
    Alzheimer's disease/dementia
        173–4
    blood clots 167–70

breast cancer risk 161–7
Chinese herbal medicine compared
    with 87–8
colorectal cancer 159
controversy around 154
dehydroepiandrosterone (DHEA)
    184–5
diabetes 159
different methods of taking 178
different types and risk 165–6
duration of use and risk 162–3
endometrial cancer 173
gallbladder disease 171
heart health 158–9, 167–71
history of 151–4
how long to take for 177
and life expectancy 174
lung cancer 173
migraines 156
new guidelines published 147
oestrogen 178–9, 185–6
osteoporosis 157
ovarian cancer 172–3
overview of 148, 223–4
phytoestrogens compared with 78–9
progestogens 179–82, 186
risks overview 159–60
and sleep 139
stopping 177
stroke risk 170
testosterone 183–4
urinary tract infections 155–156,
    179, 224
vaginal dryness 155–6
when to start 177
Women's Health Initiative (WHI)
    study 153, 154, 163–5
    see also bioidentical hormone
        replacement therapy (BHRT)
hormones
    overview of role of 16
    see also Hormone Replacement
        Therapy (HRT)
hot flushes
    CBT for 94–5
    Clonidine 204–5
    dietary supplements 72–3
    evening primrose oil 82–3
    Gabapentin 203–4
    hypnotherapy for 98–9

hot flushes *cont*
  overview of 22
  red clover 77
  SNRIs 203
  SSRIs 202
hyperthyroidism 215
hypnotherapy 96–9, 104–7
hypoactive sexual desire disorder
  (HSDD) 183–4
hypothyroidism 214

Intrauterine system (IUS) 182–3
invisible, becoming 42–3

Ketogenic diet 53
Kupperman index 72

libido loss 23
life expectancy and HRT 174
low-fat foods 132
lung cancer 173

medical help, when to seek 28
medical management
  Clonidine 204–5
  Gabapentin 203–4
  SERMS (selective oestrogen
    receptor modulators) 199–201
  SNRIs (serotonin-norepinephrine
    reuptake inhibitors) 203
  SSRIs (selective serotonin reuptake
    inhibitors) 202
  Tibolone 197–9
Mediterranean style diet 60
memory loss 32–4, 86, 173–4
Menopausal Hormone Therapy *see*
  Hormone Replacement Therapy
  (HRT)
menopause
  premature 19–20, 181–2
  reason for 14
menstrual cycle
  anovulatory cycles 21
  overview of 15–6
migraines 24–6, 62, 156

mind-body medicine *see*
  complementary and alternative
  medicine (CAM) therapies
mindfulness-based stress reduction
  (MBSR) 100
Mirena coil 182–3

napping 137–8
night sweats 23, 94–95, 138, 155 197
  222
nutrition *see* diet; dietary supplements

oestradiol (E2) 18, 178, 190
oestriol (E3) 19, 178, 190
Oestrogel 188
oestrogen
  in bioidentical hormone
    replacement therapy (BHRT)
    187–8
  in Hormone Replacement Therapy
    (HRT) 178–9, 185–6
  overview of role of 18–9
  receptors 190–1
  selective oestrogen receptor
    modulators (SERMS) 199–201
oestrone (E1) 18, 178
omega oils 52
online support groups 143
osteoporosis
  bisphosphonates (BPs) for 206–9,
    211–2
  bone health advice 225–6
  calcium and 79–82
  HRT and 157
  overview of 30–1
  parathyroid hormone (PTH) 211
  possible over-diagnosis of 209–11
  red clover for 78
  risk factors 30–1
ovarian cancer 172–3

pain during intercourse (dyspareunia)
  23, 155–156, 179, 200
palpitations, heart 26
parathyroid hormone (PTH) 211
perfluorochemicals (PFCs) 20, 64
perimenopause 14, 21–2, 181
pesticides 64

phytoestrogens 71–9
placebo effect 73–4
plastic bottles 65–6
positive aspects
  improved sex life 44, 45
  increased confidence 45–6
  more freedom 46–7
  relief from menstruation 43–4
Premarin 151, 152, 153, 186
premature menopause 19–20, 181–2
premature ovarian insufficiency (POI)
  20, 181, 194, 223
processed meat 50–1
Prochieve 188
progesterone
  in bioidentical hormone
    replacement therapy (BHRT)
    188–9
  in Hormone Replacement Therapy
    (HRT) 179–82, 186
  overview of role of 19
Promensil 77
Prometrium 188
psychological factors
  becoming invisible 42–3
  body image 41–3, 45
psychological/behavioural therapies
  British Psychological Society
    regulation 102–3
  cognitive behavioural therapy
    (CBT) 92–6, 102–4
  finding a qualified therapist 101–7
  Health and Care Professions
    Council (HCPC) 103–4
  helps physical symptoms 91–2
  hypnotherapy 96–9, 104–7
  mindfulness-based stress reduction
    (MBSR) 100
  questions to ask prospective
    therapist 106
  relaxation training 101
psychoneuroimmunology (PNI) 91–2
pyjamas, wicking 138

raloxifene 200
red clover 77–8
red meat 50
reflexology 115–7

relationship issues
  educating your partner 140–1
  see also sex life
relaxation training 101
Rimostil 77

St John's wort 85–6
salt intake 51
saturated fat 53
selective oestrogen receptor
  modulators (SERMS) 199–201
selective serotonin reuptake inhibitors
  (SSRIs) 202
sequential combined regimen 181
SERMS (selective oestrogen receptor
  modulators) 199–201
serotonin-norepinephrine reuptake
  inhibitors (SNRIs) 203
17beta-oestradiol 187–8, 190
sex life
  discussions with partner 141–2
  hypoactive sexual desire disorder
    (HSDD) 183–4
  improvement in 44, 45
  libido loss 23
  testosterone and 183–4
  see also vaginal dryness
sleep
  alcohol and 137
  breathing exercises for better 139
  depression and 139
  devices and 135–6
  general sleep hygiene 135–8
  HRT and 139
  insomnia 27
  menopause-specific symptoms
    138–9
  napping 137–8
  noise and 136
  reflexology for 117
  room temperature 138
  wicking pyjamas 138
sleep apnoea 27
SNRIs (serotonin-norepinephrine
  reuptake inhibitors) 203
social support
  and health 142–3
  online support groups 143

Somers, Suzanne 149–50
soya 71–6
spirits (alcohol) 61
SSRIs (selective serotonin reuptake
    inhibitors) 202
stress *see* psychological factors;
    psychological/behavioural
    therapies
stroke 170
sugar 54
supplements *see* dietary supplements
surfactants 64
symptom diary 127–31

tai chi 119–20
tamoxifen 75, 200
testing
    2-OHE:16 alpha-OHE1 ratio 215–6
    blood vs. saliva 213
    homocysteine 216–8
    measuring stress hormones 213–4
    overview of 212–3
    thyroid tests 214–5
    urine tests 215–6
    vaginal ultrasound scans 216
testosterone 183–4, 189
therapists
    British Psychological Society
        regulation 102–3
    cognitive behavioural therapists
        102–4
    complaints 105, 122
    Complementary and Natural
        Healthcare Council (CNHC)
        register 122
    finding qualified psychotherapist
        101–7
    finding reputable complementary
        medicine therapist 121–4
    Health and Care Professions
        Council (HCPC) 103–4
    hypnotherapists 104–7
    questions to ask prospective 106,
        122–4
thyroid function
    soya and 76–7
    testing 214–5
Tibolone 197–9

triggers, identifying symptom 126–31
Type 2 diabetes 38–40, 159

urinary tract symptoms
    increased frequency 23, 155–156
    urinary incontinence 23, 155–156
    urinary tract infections 23, 39,
        155–156, 179, 197, 215, 224
urogenital atrophy 23, 155–156,
    see also urinary tract symptoms
Utrogestan 188

vaginal dryness
    HRT for 155–6
    lubricants/moisturisers for 205–6
    see also pain during intercourse
        (dyspareunia)
vaginal ultrasound scans 216
vegetables 58–9
venous thromboembolism (VTE)
    167–70
vitamin D 79–82
vitamin K 82
Vivelle 188

walking 134–5
water filters 66
weight
    management of 131–3
    World Cancer Research Fund
        recommendations 50
wicking pyjamas 138
wild yam extract 186
Wiley Protocol 149–50
wine 61
Women's Health Initiative (WHI)
    study 153, 154, 163–5
World Cancer Research Fund
    recommendations 49–53

yam extract 186
yoga 111–3